How Dangerous Are Performance-Enhancing Drugs?

Lydia Bjornlund

INCONTROVERSY

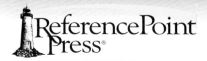

ReferencePoint
Press®

San Diego, CA

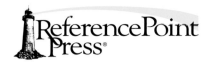

© 2011 ReferencePoint Press, Inc.

For more information, contact:
ReferencePoint Press, Inc.
PO Box 27779
San Diego, CA 92198
www.ReferencePointPress.com

Picture credits:
Cover: iStockphoto.com
Maury Aaseng: 27
AP Images: 8, 17, 19, 41, 46, 55, 63, 67, 70, 74
iStockphoto.com: 13
Landov: 33

LIBRARY OF CONGRESS CATALOGING-IN-PUBLICATION DATA

Bjornlund, Lydia D.
  How dangerous are performance-enhancing drugs? / by Lydia Bjornlund.
    p. cm. — (In controversy)
  Includes bibliographical references and index.
  ISBN-13: 978-1-60152-126-2 (hardback)
  ISBN-10: 1-60152-126-X (hardback)
  1. Anabolic steroids—Health aspects—Popular works. 2. Doping in sports—Popular works.
  3. Drug abuse—Prevention—Popular works. I. Title.
  RC1230.B56 2011
  362.29—dc22
                                                          2010017131

Contents

Foreword

I n 2008, as the U.S. economy and economies worldwide were falling into the worst recession since the Great Depression, most Americans had difficulty comprehending the complexity, magnitude, and scope of what was happening. As is often the case with a complex, controversial issue such as this historic global economic recession, looking at the problem as a whole can be overwhelming and often does not lead to understanding. One way to better comprehend such a large issue or event is to break it into smaller parts. The intricacies of global economic recession may be difficult to understand, but one can gain insight by instead beginning with an individual contributing factor such as the real estate market. When examined through a narrower lens, complex issues become clearer and easier to evaluate.

This is the idea behind ReferencePoint Press's *In Controversy* series. The series examines the complex, controversial issues of the day by breaking them into smaller pieces. Rather than looking at the stem cell research debate as a whole, a title would examine an important aspect of the debate such as *Is Stem Cell Research Necessary?* or *Is Embryonic Stem Cell Research Ethical?* By studying the central issues of the debate individually, researchers gain a more solid and focused understanding of the topic as a whole.

Each book in the series provides a clear, insightful discussion of the issues, integrating facts and a variety of contrasting opinions for a solid, balanced perspective. Personal accounts and direct quotes from academic and professional experts, advocacy groups, politicians, and others enhance the narrative. Sidebars add depth to the discussion by expanding on important ideas and events. For quick reference, a list of key facts concludes every chapter. Source notes, an annotated organizations list, bibliography, and index provide student researchers with additional tools for papers and class discussion.

The *In Controversy* series also challenges students to think critically about issues, to improve their problem-solving skills, and to sharpen their ability to form educated opinions. As President Barack Obama stated in a March 2009 speech, success in the twenty-first century will not be measurable merely by students' ability to "fill in a bubble on a test but whether they possess 21st century skills like problem-solving and critical thinking and entrepreneurship and creativity." Those who possess these skills will have a strong foundation for whatever lies ahead.

No one can know for certain what sort of world awaits today's students. What we can assume, however, is that those who are inquisitive about a wide range of issues; open-minded to divergent views; aware of bias and opinion; and able to reason, reflect, and reconsider will be best prepared for the future. As the international development organization Oxfam notes, "Today's young people will grow up to be the citizens of the future: but what that future holds for them is uncertain. We can be quite confident, however, that they will be faced with decisions about a wide range of issues on which people have differing, contradictory views. If they are to develop as global citizens all young people should have the opportunity to engage with these controversial issues."

In Controversy helps today's students better prepare for tomorrow. An understanding of the complex issues that drive our world and the ability to think critically about them are essential components of contributing, competing, and succeeding in the twenty-first century.

A Growing Controversy

When 17-year-old Matthew Dear became ill in April 2009, his parents thought he had food poisoning from the previous day's barbecue. He had been sick for about a week when his condition took a drastic turn for the worse. "He said he didn't know where he was," said his father. "His pupils were the size of saucers and he seemed really ill. When the paramedics arrived, Matt told them he'd taken steroids."[1] This was the first his father had heard about Matt's steroid use.

For most of his teenage years, Matthew Dear had dreamed of becoming a member of Great Britain's elite armed forces. To prepare, he spent hours in the gym and refused to take painkillers or eat chocolate, which he thought would undermine his fitness. Dear also took anabolic steroids, a synthetic hormone used to increase muscle mass and strength. (According to the National Institute on Drug Abuse, the proper name for the category of drugs used to build muscles is anabolic/androgenic steroids, but they are commonly referred to simply as anabolic steroids. This book uses the term *anabolic steroids* or simply *steroids* to refer to this group of drugs.)

In the hospital, Matthew Dear seemed to rebound. He was released but was readmitted within a day after he suddenly lost his eyesight. Dear died on April 20, 2009, just three months before he was to take his armed forces test. An autopsy showed swelling in his brain.

News of Matthew Dear's death created a sensation in Britain. His parents used his death to warn people of the dangers of using anabolic steroids. "He was such a good kid—pure gold," said Matthew's father. "He lived for joining the armed forces. But our healthy, strong son fell to pieces before our eyes because he took steroids."[2] His mother added, "We just hope that by sharing our pain over his tragic death we can help save someone else's life and make them think twice about taking steroids."[3]

Building Muscle and Endurance

Anabolic steroids like those Matthew Dear took are the most common group of drugs taken to enhance strength or endurance. Anabolic (meaning muscle-building) steroids are synthetic drugs that are designed to replicate testosterone, a hormone that is found naturally in the body and tells the body to grow muscle. In men, most testosterone is produced in the testicles, but it is produced in much lower levels by the adrenal glands in both males and females. Synthetic steroids are taken in much larger doses than are found naturally in the body.

Users of anabolic steroids sometimes take them in conjunction with human growth hormone (hGH). Although growth hormones have been banned by most athletic organizations, experts believe an increasing number of athletes have used hGH since the 1990s. Because hGH occurs naturally in the human body, it is difficult to detect; the first known case of an athlete illegally using the drug occurred in 2010.

Athletes also have sought to increase energy and endurance by increasing the amount of oxygen in the blood. They may inject a synthetic form of erythropoietin (EPO), which acts on stem cells in the bone marrow to increase the production of red blood cells. Athletes have also used blood transfusions of oxygenated blood—a method commonly referred to as blood doping.

Amphetamines are another class of performance-enhancing drugs. Amphetamines stimulate the brain areas associated with vigilance, mood, and alertness by releasing norepinephrine, a substance stored in nerve endings. Norepinephrine tells the body to speed up the heart and the metabolism. Athletic organizers have banned many amphetamines, although coffee and other caffeine products are often exempt. Cyclists, runners, and other endurance athletes sometimes take legal or illegal amphetamines

"Our healthy, strong son fell to pieces before our eyes because he took steroids."[2]

— Chris Dear, father of Matthew Dear, who died at 17.

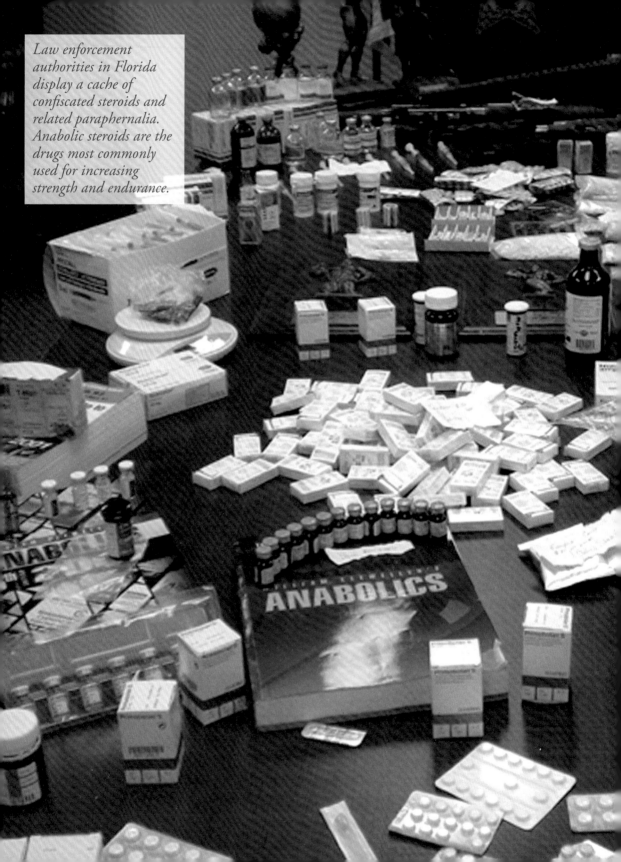

Law enforcement authorities in Florida display a cache of confiscated steroids and related paraphernalia. Anabolic steroids are the drugs most commonly used for increasing strength and endurance.

to give them a short-term surge of physical strength and mental alertness.

Diuretics, which increase the frequency of urination, are also used illicitly in many sports to artificially speed the loss of weight. Jockeys, gymnasts, and dancers are among the groups that sometimes use diuretics. Boxers and wrestlers also might use diuretics so they drop enough weight to compete in a lower weight class. Diuretics can also be used to mask the use of other banned substances.

Performance-Enhancing Drugs Today

Experts disagree about the risks involved in using performance-enhancing drugs and the ethics of their use in athletic competition. Some experts warn that athletes at any level may feel they need to take a drug to be competitive. Thomas H. Murray, president of the Hastings Center, an independent think tank on social policy, is among those who worry about the impact:

> Sports that revere records and historical comparisons (think of baseball and home runs) would become un-moored by drug-aided athletes obliterating old standards. Athletes, caught in the sport arms race, would be pressed to take more and more drugs, in ever wilder combinations and at increasingly higher doses. The drug race in sport has the potential to create a slow-motion public health catastrophe.[4]

While much of the debate has centered on the prevalence of performance-enhancing drugs in professional sports and the Olympics, the use of performance-enhancing drugs has spread beyond elite athletes. Athletes in college, high school, and even younger are sometimes tempted to take drugs to gain a competitive edge. Experts caution that the health risks for people who are still growing are greater than for adults.

Using steroids or other drugs without a prescription from a licensed physician amounts to drug abuse. It is illegal. And, as seen in the case of Matthew Dear, it can be deadly.

"The drug race in sport has the potential to create a slow-motion public health catastrophe."[4]

— Thomas H. Murray, president of the Hastings Center.

Facts

- More than 100 different types of anabolic steroids have been developed, but only a few have been approved for use by humans or animals. In the United States steroids require a prescription.

- Most synthetic anabolic steroids have 100 times as much testosterone as is produced naturally by an adult male. This is 2,000 times as much as is found naturally in a woman's body.

- Experts at the Center for Substance Abuse Research estimate that over $400 million of steroids are sold on the black market each year.

- According to the U.S. Drug Enforcement Administration, more than 1 million Americans—or 0.5 percent of the adult population—have abused anabolic steroids.

- Athletes at all levels are growing in size. For instance, the average player on Michigan State University's football team in 1975 weighed 213 pounds (96.6kg); the average weight in 2005 was 236 pounds (107kg). Experts suggest that the weight gain among football players at all levels is due to the widespread use of anabolic steroids.

What Are the Origins of the Performance-Enhancing Drugs Controversy?

The practice of using substances to enhance performance has gone on since people first started competing athletically. As early as 776 B.C., athletes used mushrooms, herbs, and spirits to enhance alertness, agility, or strength. In Greece, Olympians ate crushed sheep testicles as a means to boost testosterone levels. Roman gladiators took hallucinogens and stimulants such as strychnine to stave off fatigue. In ancient civilizations of South America, athletes chewed coca leaves—from which cocaine is derived—to make them more alert and stave off pain.

Experts say that athletes also used performance-enhancing drugs in the early modern Olympics and other international sporting events. An article published by the World Psychiatric Association says that performance-enhancing drugs were common in sports a century ago: "Mixtures of strychnine, heroin, cocaine, and caffeine were used widely by athletes and each coach or team developed its own unique secret formulae. This was common practice until heroin and cocaine became available only by prescription in the 1920s."[5]

11

Athletes often took performance-enhancing drugs despite their known risks. Marathon runner Thomas Hicks used a mixture of brandy and strychnine to improve his performance at the 1904 Olympics—a mixture that nearly killed him. Strychnine, a stimulant that is fatal in high doses, is a common ingredient in rat poison today. Meanwhile, cyclers on the grueling three-week Tour de France competition routinely added caffeine, peppermint, cocaine, and strychnine to their coffee or brandy. Cyclists also were given nitroglycerin to ease breathing after sprints. "For as long as the Tour has existed, since 1903, its participants have been doping themselves. No dope, no hope," says Hans Halter, a German journalist and physician. "The Tour, in fact, is only possible because—not despite the fact—there is doping."[6]

Early Controversy Leads to Bans

Controversy over performance-enhancing drugs escalated in the mid-1950s, when the Olympics and other worldwide competitions raised questions about the dominance of some countries. The USSR bodybuilders and weight-lifting teams dominated their events at the 1952 Olympics in Helsinki and the 1954 World Weightlifting Championships. A doctor working for the Soviet team admitted that the athletes had been given testosterone injections, which at the time was not against the rules. During the next 20 years, East German athletes rose to prominence as an Olympic powerhouse, causing judges, organizers, and spectators to wonder whether they, too, were taking steroids.

Performance-enhancing drugs continued to be used in other sports as well. Cyclists and long-distance runners often depended on stimulants to keep up their energy. At the 1960 Olympic Games in Rome, Danish cyclist Knud Enemark Jensen collapsed during a race and later died. An autopsy showed that he was under the influence of amphetamines, which had caused him to lose consciousness. Just seven years later, British cyclist Tom Simpson collapsed and died during the Tour de France. His death was attributed to heart failure induced by amphetamines.

Studies confirmed concerns about the medical risks associated with the use of performance-enhancing drugs, and sports organizations began to ban their use. In 1963 France became the first country to enact an anti-doping law. Other countries followed suit, as did the International Cycling Union, which governs the Tour de France and other world cycling events, and the Fédération Internationale de Football Association (FIFA), which oversees the World Cup soccer tournament.

In 1967 the International Olympic Committee (IOC), which oversees the Olympic events, established a list of prohibited substances. The IOC began to test athletes for doping—the use of performance-enhancing drugs—at the 1972 Olympics at Munich. The IOC added anabolic steroids to the list of banned substances and methods in 1975 and began testing athletes for steroid use at the 1976 Olympic Games in Montreal.

Performance-Enhancing Drugs at the Olympics

By then it was clear that doping worked. Olympic athletes saw that the use of performance-enhancing drugs could help in the quest for a medal. Athletes—often with the help of their coaches,

Steroid use is rampant among bodybuilders. Controversy over performance-enhancing drugs in the 1950s brought attention, in particular, to Olympic bodybuilders and weightlifters from the former Soviet Union.

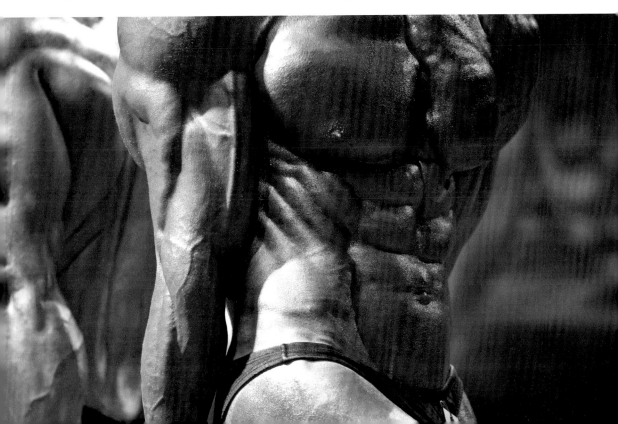

Beyond Athletics

Much of the controversy around performance-enhancing drugs is focused on sports, but athletes are not the only people who use performance-enhancing drugs. Body-builders and others who seek a "ripped" appearance often rely on anabolic steroids to bulk up. Performance-enhancing drugs also are common in the entertainment industry. Models, actors, musicians, dancers, and other performers may use drugs to overcome stage fright, improve their bodies, strengthen their voice, or give them more stamina. One source estimates that one-third of rappers use steroids and hGH to get the ripped appearance that appeals to record labels and fans. A prominent Hollywood plastic surgeon asserts, "If you're an actor in Hollywood and you're over 40, you are doing hGH. Period. Why wouldn't you? It makes your skin look better, your hair, your fingernails, everything."

Quoted in Jack McCallum, "The Real Dope," *SI.com*, March 11, 2008, p 2. http://sportsillustrated.cnn.com.

trainers, and doctors—continued to use performance-enhancing drugs. Some looked for alternatives to the list of drugs that were banned; researchers could develop new steroids by changing the molecular structure of a banned drug. When these alternatives could not be found, athletes took the drugs surreptitiously and found ingenious ways to beat the testing programs.

Drug use was difficult to prove. In the 1970s some Olympic competitors suspected drug use among the East German women's swimming team. The muscles of the swimmers bulged; their voices were deeper than usual. At the 1976 Olympics in Montreal, East German women swimmers won 11 of the 13 individual gold medals, setting 8 world records in the process. American swimmer Shirley Babashoff, a gold-medal hopeful, complained at the time of cheating among the East Germans. "They had gotten so big, and when we heard their voices, we thought we were in a coed locker room," she recalled in 2004. "I don't know why it wasn't obvious to other people, too."[7] Babashoff lost several races to the East German swimmers, and her criticisms were cast aside as sour grapes by Olympic organizers and the media.

Classified documents released after the fall of the Berlin Wall confirmed Babashoff's claims. The swimmers themselves have since spoken out about the drugs, claiming a range of health problems including liver tumors, heart disease, cancer, infertility, and depression. Two of the athletes also claim that the drugs led to birth defects among their children. In 2000 several of these women testified at the trial of Lothar Kipke, the former chief doctor of East Germany's swimming team, who was convicted of giving anabolic steroids to the women without their knowledge.

While steroids were common among those seeking strength, participants in marathons, cycling, cross-country skiing, and other endurance events continued to look for ways to increase their supply of oxygen by boosting their red blood cell counts. Some athletes sought to accomplish this by removing their own blood, storing it, and transfusing it back just before a race. In the early 1980s scientists figured out how to manufacture a synthetic form of erythropoietin (EPO), the hormone that stimulates the formation of red blood cells. After the 1984 Olympic Games, the IOC, the National Collegiate Athletic Association, and the American College of Sports Medicine issued a ruling that "any blood doping procedure used in an attempt to improve athletic performance is unethical, unfair, and exposes the athlete to unwarranted and potentially serious health risks."[8]

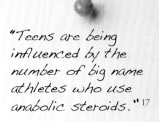

"Teens are being influenced by the number of big name athletes who use anabolic steroids." [17]

— Kristie Leong, family physician and health and wellness writer.

Catching Cheaters

As the risks of drug use became known, sports organizations began to ban their use. At the 1968 Olympic Games, Sweden's Hans-Gunnar Liljenwall earned the dubious distinction of becoming the first Olympic athlete to test positive for using a banned substance. Liljenwall was stripped of the bronze medal he had won in the pentathlon. In 1972 Olympic swimmer Rick DeMont became the first American caught taking ephedrine, a stimulant that was on the list of banned substances.

Perhaps the most memorable case of cheating at the Olympic Games involved Canadian sprinter Ben Johnson. Johnson won the 100-meter sprint at the 1988 Seoul Olympics with a world record–breaking time, but he was stripped of the gold medal after his urine tested positive for stanazalol, a steroid that was on the list of banned substances. Johnson was banned from competition for two years. In 1993 he again tested positive for drugs and was permanently banned from competition.

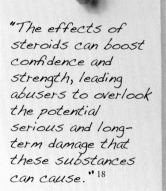

"The effects of steroids can boost confidence and strength, leading abusers to overlook the potential serious and long-term damage that these substances can cause." [18]

— Nora D. Volkow, director of the National Institute on Drug Abuse.

The IOC simply could not keep pace with the growing use of performance-enhancing drugs. Their use expanded from one sport to another, one country to another. "Through the 1980s and 1990s, clandestine doping programs spread from sport to sport guided by modern, albeit unethical, pharmacists and sports medicine professionals,"[9] write researchers David A. Baron, David M. Martin, and Samir Abol Magd in a 2007 article reviewing the growth of performance-enhancing drugs worldwide. Robert Kerr, a California physician, later admitted to providing steroids to 3,000 to 4,000 patients, many of whom he said were celebrities and athletes. Among them, according to Kerr, were 20 medal winners in the 1984 Olympics. He was not alone. Baron, Martin, and Magd explain, "Doping became so prevalent in Olympic sport that some argued that all records should be discarded or put on hold until all forms of doping could be detected and stopped."[10]

In the past several years, catching cheaters has become increasingly difficult. In 2002 scientists began experimenting with a new group of synthetic steroids designed to be undetectable by drug tests. These so-called "designer" steroids are intended for use by athletes and have no approved medical use. Because they have not been approved (in any dose) by the U.S. Food and Drug Administration (FDA), some experts say they have far greater risks than the drugs that came before them.

Cycling

Olympic athletes were not alone in their quest to improve performance through the use of drugs. For decades, allegations of doping have plagued the Tour de France. John Hoberman, a doping historian who has written several books on the topic, writes:

> Cycling has been the most consistently drug-soaked major sport of the 20th and 21st centuries. While weightlifting and shot-putting have also been thoroughly drug-dependent, they are minor cults compared with the cycling carnival that plays across Europe every year. . . . Over the past 50 years, a majority of Tour champions as well as second- and third-place finishers have been confirmed or accused dopers at some point in their careers.[11]

In 1998 alleged drug use took center stage during the race when large quantities of doping products were found in the car of France's Festina cycling team. The members of the Festina team were arrested and ejected from the race. Police raids also uncovered

Canadian sprinter Ben Johnson (right) turns in a record-breaking win during the 1988 Seoul Olympics 100-meter dash. Johnson was later stripped of his gold medal and banned from competition after testing positive for a banned substance.

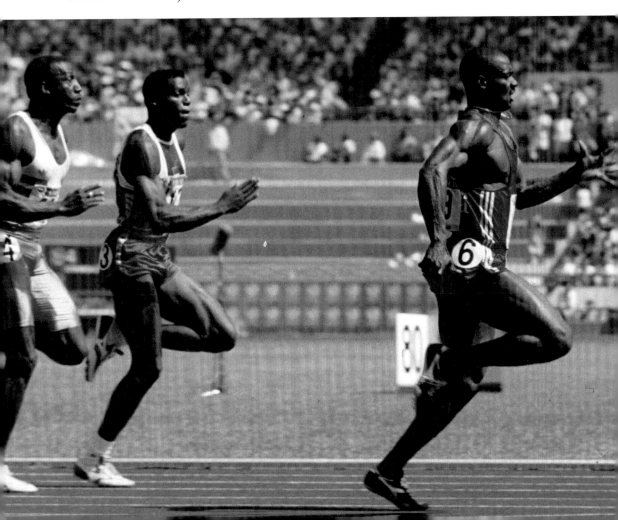

drugs in the rooms of the Dutch TVM team. The doping scandal caused numerous riders to drop out. Only 14 of the 21 teams that began the race—and 96 of the 189 riders—finished. Experts suspect that most, if not all, of these riders would have tested positive for banned substances.

The 1998 raids caused a scandal among the media and spectators, but participants say everyone involved in the race knew about the widespread use of performance-enhancing drugs. Swiss rider Alex Zülle explains how the cover-up of the doping culture worked:

> I've been in this business for a long time. I know what goes on. And not just me, everyone knows. The riders, the team leaders, the organizers, the officials, the journalists. As a rider you feel tied into this system. It's like being on the highway. The law says there's a speed limit of 65, but everyone is driving 70 or faster. Why should I be the one who obeys the speed limit? So I had two alternatives: either fit in and go along with the others or go back to being a house painter. And who in my situation would have done that?[12]

Many cyclists have since admitted to using EPO and other performance enhancers during their cycling careers. In 2010, the 2006 Tour de France champion Floyd Landis admitted to using numerous banned substances during his career, including testosterone patches, human growth hormone, and EPO. Landis, who repeatedly denied using performance-enhancing drugs until making his surprise admission, was officially stripped of his title in 2007 after failing a drug test.

Scandal in Professional Sports

In professional sports in the United States, the controversy over the use of performance-enhancing drugs dates back to the 1980s, when concerns were first raised about the use of steroids among football, baseball, and other professional athletes.

Suspicions were heightened in the late 1990s, when sportswriters mused openly about whether the race to beat Major League Baseball's long-standing home-run record set by Roger Maris was fueled by steroids. In 1998 Sammy Sosa and Mark McGwire matched homerun for homerun, resulting in a record-breaking season in which both players surpassed Maris's record. Both Sosa and McGwire denied using drugs to enhance their performance. In early 2010—more than a decade later—McGwire admitted that he had used anabolic steroids. Although he apologized for his use of steroids, he reiterated earlier comments that he began using steroids to heal from injury, not to improve his home-run performance or batting average.

By the early 2000s there was growing evidence that the use of steroids and other performance-enhancing drugs was a problem among professional athletes. The players themselves began to admit that many colleagues were using drugs. In 2002 baseball player Ken Caminiti claimed that at least 50 percent of major league players used steroids. In his 2005 book José Canseco upped this figure to 85 percent. Baseball was not the only sport under attack. In a 2009 survey, almost 1 in 10 retired National Football League

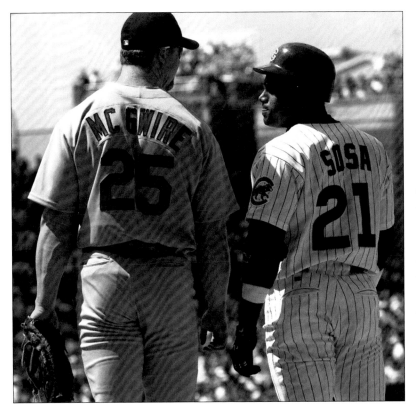

Sportswriters mused openly about steroid use in the 1990s as baseball hitting legends Mark McGwire and Sammy Sosa fought to outhit each other and beat Roger Maris's long-standing home-run record. McGwire later admitted to using steroids; Sosa has denied using them.

(NFL) players polled said they had used anabolic steroids while still playing. The numbers of steroid users were higher among football players who depended on size and strength: 16.3 percent of offensive linemen and 14.8 percent of defensive linemen admitted using steroids before the drug ban. In 2010 Dick Pound, a Canadian member of the IOC and of the World Anti-Doping Agency (WADA), estimated that more than 30 percent of National Hockey League players used performance-enhancing drugs.

In 2003 the U.S. Anti-Doping Agency worked with federal agents after receiving an anonymous tip about THG, a new synthetic steroid that athletes called "the clear" because it could not be detected. Federal agents raided the facilities of the Bay Area Laboratory Co-operative (BALCO), the alleged manufacturer of the drug. In addition to evidence of steroids and growth hormones, the agents found a list of BALCO customers. Among them were several prominent professional baseball players, NFL players, and Olympic athletes.

Major League Baseball responded by instituting its first mandatory drug-testing program, with severe penalties for those who broke the rules. Meanwhile, Congress held hearings to see whether laws banning steroids and other performance-enhancing drugs were needed.

Gene Doping: The Wave of the Future?

Some experts warn that gene doping is the danger of the future. WADA, an independent organization established in 1999 to address the use of drugs among athletes, defines gene doping as "the transfer of cells or genetic elements (e.g. DNA, RNA) [or] the use of pharmacalogical or biological agents that alter gene expression."[13] Gene doping builds on gene therapy, in which researchers have found ways to modify genes to prevent or treat serious medical conditions. The science of gene transfer makes it possible to put synthetic genes into human cells, where they become indistinguishable from a person's own DNA. This makes it possible for athletes and others to receive genes that can slow muscle atrophy, speed up the body's metabolism, or augment muscle performance.

The first product to be associated with gene doping emerged in 2006, when German authorities caught an athletic coach trying to make an online purchase of Repoxygen, a gene therapy material designed to produce EPO. Scientists know of 187 genes linked to fitness and athleticism, and experts say they could parlay this knowledge into a product used to build muscle, increase endurance, or otherwise boost performance. Although there are no known cases of gene doping, Theodore Friedmann, the head of WADA's gene doping panel, warns that "with the improvement in the gene therapy technology, the extension to sport is becoming more and more inevitable."[14]

A Drug Culture

Major League Baseball has been the subject of several "tell-all" books that claim that the use of steroids is widespread among the league's players. Books such as José Canseco's *Juiced: Wild Times, Rampant 'Roids, Smash Hits, and How Baseball Got Big* have led sportswriters and fans to scrutinize almost any athletic achievement for signs of performance enhancers. Rumors of drug use followed home-run slugger Barry Bonds for years before he hit his seven hundred fifty-sixth home run in 2007 to break Hank Aaron's record. When he reached that milestone, and even afterwards, Bonds's accomplishments on the field were questioned. Bonds vehemently defended his record. Bonds said, "This record is not tainted at all. At all. Period."[15]

"We allow people to do far more dangerous things than play football or baseball while using steroids. We allow people to . . . eat marbled meat or ice cream pie every day if they want." [20]

— Norman Fost, doctor and professor of medical ethics at the University of Wisconsin.

In response to the scandals, Congress initiated an independent investigation into the use of steroids. After a 20-month investigation led by Senator George Mitchell, Congress released its findings in 2007. The Mitchell Report detailed a deep-rooted drug culture within Major League Baseball and listed 89 players suspected of using performance-enhancing drugs, including all-stars Roger Clemens and Andy Pettitte. Baseball commissioner Bud Selig said the report was a "call to action"[16] for Major League Baseball.

Use Among Teens

As word of use among elite athletes made front-page news, people began to wonder about the influence on young people. "It seems that teens are being influenced by the number of big name athletes who use anabolic steroids," writes Dr. Kristie Leong. "Seeing their favorite sports heroes using anabolic steroids makes it look okay—even glamorous."[17]

Although many people worry that young people will follow in the footsteps of their favorite athletes, studies suggest that the use of steroids among teens is declining. The Monitoring the Future study, an annual survey funded by the National Institute on Drug Abuse, shows that the use of steroids among high school seniors is at its lowest level since 1997.

Still, any use of drugs among young people is of concern to experts. Anabolic steroids have a more profound effect on young people—and potentially permanent negative side effects. Lured by a desire to "look buff," make the team, or win an athletic scholarship, young people may ignore the risks of performance-enhancing drugs. Nora D. Volkow, the director of the National Institute on Drug Abuse, writes about anabolic steroids:

> Abuse of anabolic steroids differs from the abuse of other illicit substances because the initial abuse of anabolic steroids is not driven by the immediate euphoria that accompanies most drugs of abuse, such as cocaine, heroin, and marijuana, but by the desire of abusers to change their appearance and performance, characteristics of great importance to adolescents. The effects of steroids can boost confidence and strength, leading abusers to overlook the potential serious and long-term damage that these substances can cause.[18]

Performance-Enhancing Drugs and Elite Athletes

While most, if not all, experts agree that performance-enhancing drugs are dangerous for young people, the main controversy today revolves around the use of performance-enhancing substances among elite athletes. Some say that performance enhancers are a natural part of an athlete's will to use everything in his or her power to excel. Athletes say that performance-enhancing drugs cannot improve the skills of someone who does not have athletic

"Athletes don't take [performance-enhancing] drugs to level the playing field, they do it to get an advantage."[21]

— Dick Pound, former president of the World Anti-Doping Agency.

ability and inclination and that performance enhancers are simply one aspect of a regimen that includes hard work, diet, and exercise. "Do we want to see the highest possible achievements by men and women who do not use performance-enhancing drugs?" asks a writer for *Sports Illustrated*. "If so, what counts as performance enhancing? . . . If sports fans really want to see achievement that they can relate to, perhaps athletes should be restricted to diets of pizza and beer, and be required to have 40-hour-a-week desk jobs."[19]

Opponents of strict policies also point out that sports can be dangerous enterprises. If performance-enhancing substances improve an athlete's strength, agility, or alertness, they may actually make a sport safer. "We allow people to do far more dangerous things than play football or baseball while using steroids," points out Norman Fost, a doctor who teaches medical ethics at the University of Wisconsin. "We allow people to bungee-jump, to ski on advanced slopes, to cliff dive. To eat marbled meat or ice cream pie every day if they want."[20]

Others strenuously disagree. The dangers of performance-enhancing drugs and the unknown risks they pose require sports organizers and legislators to protect athletes, they say. Pound, the former president of WADA, suggests that athletes could become embroiled in a race in which they are encouraged to take drugs at an ever-increasing—and ever-more-dangerous—dosage. He says:

> Remember that athletes don't take these drugs to level the playing field, they do it to get an advantage. And if everyone else is doing what they're doing, then instead of taking 10 grams or 10 cc's or whatever it is, they'll take 20 or 30 or 40, and a vicious circle simply gets bigger. The end game will be an activity that is increasingly violent, extreme, and meaningless, practiced by a class of chemical and or genetic mutant gladiators.[21]

At the center of this debate are questions about whether all performance-enhancing drugs are dangerous. Those who believe that their risks do not merit making them illegal further question the fairness of prohibiting their use.

FACTS

- In 1972, prior to the International Olympic Committee's ban on anabolic steroids, 68 percent of American track and field athletes admitted to using steroids.

- More than 40 Chinese swimmers failed drug tests between 1990 and 2000, more than 3 times as many as any other nation's swim team.

- According to the 2009 Monitoring the Future study, 1.3 percent of eighth graders, 1.3 percent of tenth graders, and 2.2 percent of twelfth graders reported using steroids at least once in their lives. Statistics show a steady decline over the past five years. The high was in 2002, when 4 percent of twelfth graders reported they had used steroids.

- The Taylor Hooton Foundation reports that the median age that a student first uses anabolic steroids is 15.

- Erythropoietin is injected under the skin and can boost red blood cell count for six weeks or longer. It has been shown to increase the oxygen supply by as much as 7 to 10 percent.

- In a confidential survey, nearly 1 in 10 retired football players polled said they had used anabolic steroids while playing in the NFL.

- In a 2009 survey of retired NFL players, 16.3 percent of offensive linemen and 14.8 percent of defensive linemen admitted using steroids before they were banned.

Do Performance-Enhancing Drugs Pose a Health Risk?

Those who have spoken out against performance-enhancing drugs cite the many dangers to one's health. Studies have linked the use of some performance-enhancing drugs to cancer, heart disease, and liver and kidney damage. Risks are increased when drugs are taken at the high doses typical of users who want to enhance their performance.

Many of the steroids and other drugs that athletes use to enhance their performance have never been tested for use in humans. They may be smuggled into the country from unknown locations or made illegally in underground laboratories. And with new forms of drugs emerging each year, the longer-term health risks of the performance-enhancing drug epidemic may not be known for many decades to come.

The Medical Benefits of Performance-Enhancing Drugs

Many of the same drugs used illegally by athletes to enhance performance have legitimate uses in the treatment of all kinds of illnesses. In the mid-1930s, pharmaceutical companies began to research synthetic drugs that would replicate testosterone's healing and muscle-building powers. For the next several decades, drug companies developed and marketed several forms of testosterone-like drugs to help heal wounds, relieve the symptoms of arthritis, and treat depression.

Today steroids are prescribed to treat a wide variety of illnesses. A group of steroids called corticosteroids is a common treatment for asthma, arthritis, acne, and skin problems. The most common use of anabolic androgenic steroids—the class used by athletes and bodybuilders—is as testosterone replacement therapy for men with testicular cancer. Steroids also are often prescribed for AIDS patients to help them gain weight and defend against other diseases; to treat osteoporosis, a degenerative bone disease that can be exacerbated by low levels of testosterone; and to treat a rare form of anemia, a blood condition in which there are too few red blood cells.

Anabolic steroids also are sometimes prescribed to help people rebuild muscles after an injury requiring surgery. During the recovery process, when muscles are not used, they can shrink and weaken, or atrophy. Some athletes who have been suspected of steroid use claim that they only used the drugs as prescribed to help recovery from an illness or injury.

Under a Doctor's Care

Other drugs commonly used to enhance performance also have medical uses. In the 1930s pharmaceutical companies developed amphetamines as a nasal inhalant to treat colds and hay fever, but their uses today are primarily focused on their ability to stimulate the central nervous system. They are prescribed to treat a variety of mental disorders, narcolepsy (a disease characterized by an overwhelming urge to sleep), and alcoholism. In addition, amphetamines are used in conjunction with other drugs as a treatment for Parkinson's disease, a degenerative disorder of the central nervous system.

Many performance-enhancing drugs are safe when used as directed under a doctor's care, but experts warn that they can be extremely dangerous when used as performance enhancers. Speaking about the use of steroids, Dr. Gary Wadler, a world-renowned expert on the subject of drugs in sports, says:

> There can be a whole panoply of side effects, even with prescribed doses. Some are visible to the naked eye and

Side Effects of Steroids in Men and Women

Additional testosterone in a male's body will increase muscle mass and strength, but other, unwanted side effects will often occur. The introduction of synthetic male hormones into the body of a woman can also result in a variety of unwanted side effects.

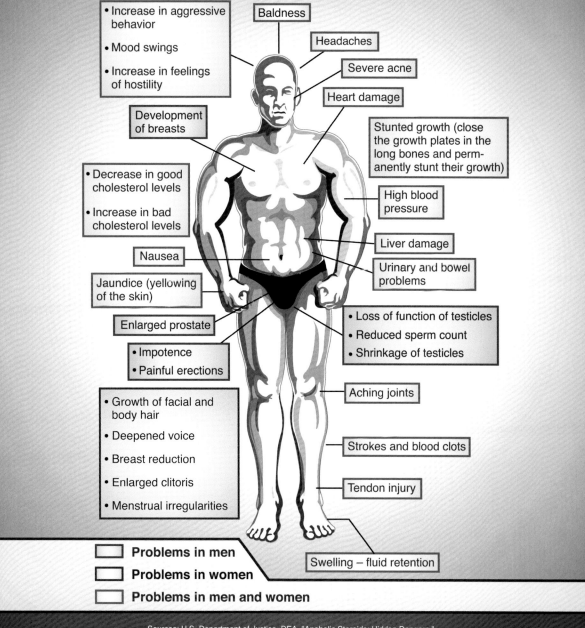

- Increase in aggressive behavior
- Mood swings
- Increase in feelings of hostility

Baldness

Headaches

Severe acne

Heart damage

Development of breasts

Stunted growth (close the growth plates in the long bones and permanently stunt their growth)

- Decrease in good cholesterol levels
- Increase in bad cholesterol levels

High blood pressure

Liver damage

Nausea

Urinary and bowel problems

Jaundice (yellowing of the skin)

Enlarged prostate

- Loss of function of testicles
- Reduced sperm count
- Shrinkage of testicles

- Impotence
- Painful erections

Aching joints

- Growth of facial and body hair
- Deepened voice
- Breast reduction
- Enlarged clitoris
- Menstrual irregularities

Strokes and blood clots

Tendon injury

Problems in men

Problems in women

Problems in men and women

Swelling – fluid retention

Sources: U.S. Department of Justice, DEA, "Anabolic Steroids: Hidden Dangers," March 2008; USA Today, "How Anabolic Steroids Work," www.usatoday.com.

some are internal. Some are physical, others are psychological. With unsupervised steroid use, wanton "megadosing" or stacking (using a combination of different steroids), the effects can be irreversible or undetected until it's too late.[22]

Athletes, bodybuilders, and others who use drugs to enhance their performance often take far higher doses than a doctor would prescribe. Those who take drugs without a prescription also may be unaware of warning signs of a dangerous side effect. Users of anabolic steroids, for instance, often fail to recognize emotional difficulties or changes in mood as a side effect of their drug use. With some drugs, the risks are heightened when users abruptly start or stop taking a drug.

Short-Term Side Effects

Although anabolic steroids help users increase muscle mass, they can have a number of negative impacts on the way one looks. Many of these effects are permanent. In men, for instance, the use of steroids sometimes results in premature baldness. Steroid abuse can lead to production of estrogen, a female hormone that regulates the growth of breasts among other things. As a result, some men grow breasts that look like women's breasts.

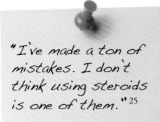

"I've made a ton of mistakes. I don't think using steroids is one of them."[25]

— Ken Caminiti, professional baseball player who was named the National League's Most Valuable Player in 1996.

In women the use of steroids makes the body more masculine. The voice deepens, thick hair grows on the face and body, and muscles bulge. Women who take steroids sometimes also experience a shrinking of the breasts and baldness. A woman's skin may thicken and darken.

Some doctors warn that steroid abuse also can lead to other, more general health problems. Steroids interfere with the body's natural system of immunity, making it more likely that users will catch common colds and flu. It may also take a steroid user longer to recover from these illnesses. Nosebleeds, headaches, stomach pain, acne, and other skin disorders are common side effects of steroid abuse. Although steroid use can have long-term negative health effects, many of these common side effects go away when the user stops taking the drug.

Gene Therapy and Doping

Gene therapy is the latest medical advance that could be abused by athletes seeking to enhance their performance. Doctors have successfully used gene therapy to replace the genes in seriously ill patients but warn that the technology is still in its infancy. Scientists have identified 187 genes linked to fitness and athleticism, and experts worry that gene therapy could result in deliberate manipulation of these genes to build muscle, increase endurance, or otherwise boost performance. In a 2010 interview Theodore Friedmann, the head of WADA's panel on gene doping, warns of the potential for abuse:

> The fact is that the material and information that the athletes have is very sparse and very incomplete and is obviously given to them with the hope of encouraging them to do something that really the science isn't ready for. And so, under those conditions, anyone who does this kind of thing really ought to be considered guilty of malpractice and certainly professional misconduct. It's dangerous. . . . In the gene therapy setting, we do these kinds of manipulations as a society, we accept [the risks] in the course of trying to do good and heal suffering—or heal illness and ease suffering. But to do the same kinds of dangerous things to healthy young athletes, I think, is really unconscionable.

Quoted in *Talk of the Nation*, "Experts: 'Gene Doping' to Be Next Sports Scandal," National Public Radio, February 5, 2010. www.npr.org.

The Impact of Steroids on Mood

Performance-enhancing drugs also can impact mood. The report of the National Institute on Drug Abuse on anabolic steroids concludes, "Although not all scientists agree, some interpret available evidence to show that anabolic steroid abuse—particularly in high doses—promotes aggression that can manifest itself as fighting, physical and sexual abuse, armed robbery, and property crimes such as burglary and vandalism."[23]

On the football field or hockey rink, aggression can be an asset, but "'roid rage" elsewhere can be dangerous. Some experts blame steroids for the mental breakdown of Chris Benoit, a professional wrestler who, over a three-day period in 2007, killed his wife and 7-year-old son before taking his own life. Toxicology reports showed 10 times the normal amount of testosterone in Benoit's system, leading some experts to speculate that steroids contributed to his rampage.

Experts also warn about the link between steroid abuse and depression. Depression is a particular danger for people withdrawing from the drug. Taylor Hooton, a pitcher on his high school baseball team in Plano, Texas, started taking steroids when he was 16 as part of an effort to gain size and strength during his senior year. He gained the size he wanted, but he also suffered from a lot of unpleasant and dangerous side effects. He developed acne on his back. He flew into rages, punching walls and pounding the floor with his fists. He started stealing things and lying to his parents. On July 15, 2003, at the age of 17, Hooton took his own life. Friends said he had stopped taking the drugs just prior to his suicide.

Not everyone agrees that anabolic steroids increase aggression, depression, or other changes in mood, however. "There is no reliable scientific data that conclusively says that elevated levels of administered testosterone lead to excessive rage or behavioral disorders," said the medical examiner following Benoit's death. "All the testing that's been done regarding that has been completely inconclusive."[24]

Serious Health Risks

The long-term use of anabolic steroids can lead to serious medical problems. Doctors warn that steroids elevate blood pressure, increase LDL cholesterol (the bad kind), and lower HDL cholesterol (the good kind). Cholesterol buildup clogs the arteries and blood vessels, which increases the risk of heart attack and stroke. Long-

"If you start making changes in your genetic makeup, who knows what you are going to trigger?"[28]

— Mark Frankel, director of the scientific freedom responsibility and law program for the American Association for the Advancement of Science.

term steroid abuse also may lead to enlargement of the heart, liver damage, and kidney failure.

Among men, large doses of steroids also cause the body to shut off its own production of testosterone. A lack of this hormone can reduce the amount of sperm a man produces, putting him at risk of infertility. Synthetic steroids also sometimes cause enlargement of the prostate gland, causing pain when urinating. Some studies also have shown a link between the use of steroids and prostate cancer, but—as with the link to other forms of cancer—the evidence is inconclusive.

Taking steroids is particularly dangerous for women. Anabolic steroids can disrupt the natural menstrual cycle and impede a woman's ability to bear children. As with so many other drugs, steroid use has special risks during pregnancy. Studies suggest that pregnant women who take even low doses of steroids are at greater risk of miscarriage. There may also be greater risk of birth defects among babies whose mothers took steroids or other performance-enhancing drugs. Several members of the East German Olympic swimming team who were given anabolic steroids during the 1970s blame the drug for birth defects in children they had many years later.

Experts cite many cases of athletes whose premature deaths may have been brought about by the use of anabolic steroids. Florence Griffith Joyner, an American sprinter who won two Olympic gold medals at the 1988 Olympics, died at just 38 from a heart seizure that experts attribute to long-term steroid use. Baseball player Ken Caminiti admitted in 2002 to having used steroids for several years, including during his MVP-winning 1996 season. Caminiti expressed no regret for his steroid use: "I've made a ton of mistakes," he said. "I don't think using steroids is one of them."[25] Still, Caminiti says he quit when his testicles "shrank to the size of peas."[26] The damage was already done. In 2004, at the age of 41, Caminiti died of a heart attack.

Dr. Eric Braverman, a cardiologist who counsels professional athletes on steroid abuse, explains that Caminiti's heart basically exploded due to years of steroid abuse. "By revving the heart up with steroids, making it grow bigger, and then taking

> "My . . . son . . . was so addicted to steroids that not even heart failure or a kidney transplant stopped him from using the drugs."[30]
>
> — Marylou Gantner, mother of a long-term steroid user who died of kidney failure at the age of 30.

those steroids away, you end up with a heart muscle that's enlarging and then contracting,"[27] he explains.

Other performance-enhancing drugs and methods also have been blamed for long-term health problems and sudden deaths. During a 2008 game in Russia's Continental Hockey League, Alexei Cherepanov, a prospect for the National Hockey League's New York Rangers, collapsed on the bench and died. Russian federal investigators ruled that Cherepanov, who reportedly died of a heart condition, had been blood doping. He was just 19 years old.

Experts also caution people about the potential dangers of gene doping, particularly on long-term health. "We basically know what steroids can do to the body," writes Mark Frankel, director of the scientific freedom responsibility and law program for the American Association for the Advancement of Science, "but at this point, we're not sure if you start making changes in your genetic makeup, who knows what you are going to trigger? Maybe it will be inert and not do even what you're hoping it will do. Or maybe it will have some unforeseen consequences for [your] health."[28]

Are the Dangers Exaggerated?

Gary Cartwright, a writer for *Texas Monthly*, is among those who believe the risks may be exaggerated. "Steroids . . . can be as benign as those that are commonly prescribed for allergies and as harmful as those that have sent many retired athletes into physical decline," he writes. "As with any medication, the effect depends on the dose and frequency of use."[29]

Doctors concede that the link between drug use and illness or death can be hard to prove. NFL player Lyle Alzado, who died from brain cancer in 1992, blamed his cancer on his longtime use of anabolic steroids. His story is repeatedly used to warn people away from steroid use, despite the fact that there is little evidence that there is any link between steroid abuse and brain tumors or any other type of cancer.

Teens at Risk

Performance-enhancing drugs—like any other substance—do not affect all people in the same way. Experts warn that they may be particularly dangerous for teens, whose bodies are not yet fully developed. Anabolic steroids, for instance, are associated with stunted growth. When the level of testosterone is higher than normal, the body stops growing. This effect is permanent; there is no way to reverse this effect of steroid use. Studies suggest that girls and women are at greater risk of the damaging effects of anabolic steroids. Whereas the bodies of males are conditioned to process testosterone, the female body produces testosterone only in very small quantities. Steroid use among young people of both sexes has also been blamed for infertility problems much later in life. There is also evidence that teens may be more susceptible to the depression, aggression, and mood swings associated with anabolic steroids. This can put them at greater risk of suicide.

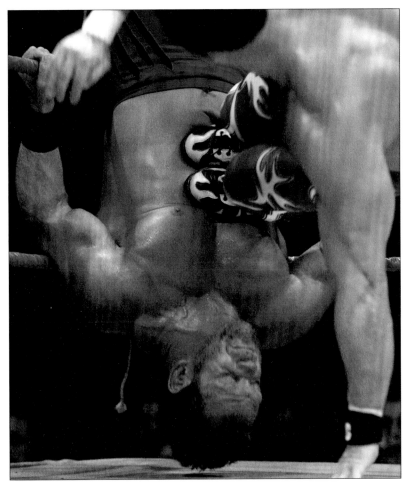

Chavo Guerrero (right) kicks Chris Benoit in the stomach during a 2006 World Wrestling Entertainment show in Spain. Benoit later committed suicide after killing his wife and young son. Experts believe steroids contributed to his rampage.

Antidrug advocates caution that teens often do not appreciate the risks involved in taking performance-enhancing drugs. Young people tend to deny their mortality—they feel as if they will live forever. Even when faced with the tragedies of others, teens tend to feel immune to danger and often take risks that more mature people would not consider. Teens also risk becoming physically and psychologically addicted to a drug, making quitting nearly impossible. Marylou Gantner, a health professional in Orlando, Florida, began to campaign against the use of steroids after her son committed suicide at the age of 30. In a book titled *Steroids Kill,* she told about her son's foray into steroids:

> He started out, I'm sure, like a lot of others do. He confided to a friend during his junior year of high school that he would use the steroids just to help him get big enough to earn a football scholarship. Then he would quit. Well, after four years of college football, followed by three years of professional football, my 6'4" nearly 300-pound son still didn't think he was big enough. He was so addicted to steroids that not even heart failure or a kidney transplant stopped him from using the drugs.[30]

Not FDA Approved

Part of the danger of performance-enhancing drugs stems from the fact that most of the drugs taken illegally have never been tested on humans or approved by the FDA, which oversees the safety of the U.S. drug supply. Some of the anabolic steroids sold to athletes and bodybuilders were designed to be used in livestock. Others are manufactured illegally. Like other illegal drugs, performance-enhancing drugs on the black market may be mixed with chalk, sugar, flour, or other ingredients that enable the dealer to make more profit. Some illegal steroids are mixed in a kitchen sink by someone following directions found on the Internet. Unhygienic conditions and the inexperience of the drug makers combine to increase the risk that the resulting compound will be contaminated with bacteria, mold, or other impurities. "If [performance-enhancing] drugs are pure, they

Creatine

Many athletes take nutritional supplements instead of or in addition to performance-enhancing drugs. Unlike anabolic steroids or other prescription drugs, many supplements are available legally as powders or pills. With annual sales of over $200 million, creatine is perhaps the most popular supplement among athletes. Creatine is a natural amino acid that provides energy to muscles. Evidence suggests that creatine may benefit athletes by producing short-term bursts of power and delaying muscle fatigue.

Some of the common side effects of creatine can interfere with its potential benefits, however. Common side effects include stomach and muscle cramps, nausea, and diarrhea. Use of creatine also may increase the risk of dehydration among athletes. Creatine appears safe for adults at doses recommended by manufacturers, but it is unknown what effect taking creatine could have over the long term, especially in young people. Experts warn that high doses of creatine could result in kidney or liver damage. Because the FDA considers supplements to be food, not drugs, the manufacturers of creatine and other supplements are not required to conform to the same safety standards as drug manufacturers. Some supplements are a mixture of elements, which has led to many instances of positive drug tests among unwitting athletes.

are dangerous," Wadler says. "If you have no idea what you're swallowing or injecting, it becomes true Russian Roulette. . . . The problem is we're not dealing with drugs from the regular marketplace."[31]

There are also risks associated with steroid injections and blood doping. Anabolic steroids are meant to be injected into a muscle; if they are accidentally injected into a vein, they can result in death. In addition, infections such as HIV and hepatitis are sometimes caused by using a needle that is not sterile.

The risks that stem from illegal drug use are among the reasons that some people advocate legalizing performance-enhancing drugs. Kate Schmidt, a U.S. Olympian who twice won the bronze medal for the javelin throw, says that allowing athletes to take drugs would make the drugs safer:

> Use could be made safer, clinical trials could be performed and dangerous overuse curbed. The technology exists to test for levels of most of the substances on the "banned drugs" lists. What if we declared that certain levels of them in the body were acceptable, while excessive amounts would result in penalties? Athletes could satisfy their drive to be faster and stronger. Drugs could move from the black market to the legitimate sports-medicine community. Athletes could stop experimenting on themselves.[32]

Addiction and Withdrawal

Experts disagree about the addictive characteristics of performance-enhancing drugs. Even when the drugs are not physically addictive, users may find it difficult to wean themselves off. Studies show that, given the choice, animals on anabolic steroids will continue using the drugs when researchers stop dosing them. People, too, often continue using steroids despite their negative physical and emotional side effects. The risks that some people take to obtain illegal drugs and the money they end up spending on them are further evidence that the drugs may be psychologically addictive.

Some performance-enhancing drugs have unpleasant side effects when the user stops using them. When a person stops using a drug, the body goes through changes. Steroid abusers may lose muscle mass, for instance. This can be very disheartening to those who have used the drug as part of an effort to look good. Some people may experience depression or loss of self-esteem as a result. Other withdrawal symptoms include sleeplessness, anxiety, fatigue, and mood swings.

Research suggests that some users turn to other drugs to alleviate some of the negative effects of performance-enhancing drugs.

They may take narcotics to counteract the effects of a stimulant or steroid, for instance. Some studies have shown a link between the use of anabolic steroids and opioids, leading experts to caution that anabolic steroids could be a gateway to hard-core drug use. While the vast majority of athletes who take steroids never turn to other drugs, the abuse of steroids themselves can undermine the health not only of athletes but also of the sports in which they participate.

FACTS

- Anabolic steroids are especially dangerous for females because the female body is not equipped to manage large doses of testosterone. Males make about 20 to 30 times as much testosterone as females do.

- In the 2009 Monitoring the Future study, 60.2 percent of twelfth graders said that anabolic steroids posed a "great risk," and 90.3 percent disapproved of the use of steroids.

- Nearly 30 percent of anabolic steroid users experience adverse effects, only some of which are reversible when the drug is stopped.

- Of 52 German athletes given anabolic steroids during the 1970s and 1980s who were examined in a 2007 study, roughly 25 percent got some form of cancer, and 33 percent reported thoughts or attempts of suicide. The risk of miscarriage and stillbirth among female athletes was 32 times higher than among the general German population.

- A 2000 study of 227 men admitted to a private treatment center for heroin and/or opioid abuse found that 9.3 percent had abused anabolic steroids before trying any other illicit drug. Of these, 86 percent first used opioids to counteract insomnia and irritability resulting from the steroids.

CHAPTER THREE

Do Performance-Enhancing Drugs Harm the Integrity of Sports?

There is no doubt that sports fans admire athletic accomplishments. The baseball player who breaks decades-old hitting records, the swimmer who consistently touches the wall hundredths of a second before his competitors, the long-distance runner who outlasts her competitors—these are the moments that bring sports to life.

In the past decade, however, these accomplishments have been overshadowed by suspicions that the athletes breaking records are doing so with the help of performance-enhancing drugs. Suspicions have intensified with each athlete who has admitted to the use of steroids or been caught using a banned substance. The prevalence of performance-enhancing drugs has raised questions about the integrity of some of the best athletes and the nature of sports and sportsmanship.

The Spirit of Sport

Many people believe that the use of performance-enhancing drugs undermines the essence of sports. Playing under the influence of drugs is simply not a part of sport, and those who take drugs are not exhibiting good sportsmanship. Winning is supposed to be the result of hard work, determination, and athleticism. Thomas H. Murray, president of the Hastings Center, argues that "natural talents and their perfection are the point of sports"[33] and that allowing the use of performance-enhancing drugs undermines these principles.

WADA argues that the use of performance-enhancing drugs "is fundamentally contrary to the spirit of sport."[34] Sport is supposed to be about honesty and integrity. Competition focuses on winning by following the rules. "[The] intrinsic value often referred to as 'the spirit of sport' . . . combines ethical notions of fairness and a level playing field with excellence in athletic performance," writes Paul C. McCaffrey, a law associate, in an article encouraging stronger antidrug measures. "The illicit use of performance-enhancing substances—commonly referred to as 'doping'—is irreconcilable with the spirit of sport."[35]

Would Legalizing Drugs Help Level the Playing Field?

Sports organizers emphasize the impact of performance enhancing drugs on fairness. In sports at any level, athletes who use performance-enhancing drugs gain an advantage over those who choose to remain clean. It is unfair when a high school football team loses the championship to a team whose players are using steroids. It is unfair when an Olympic athlete loses his or her place on the team to someone who is taking illegal substances. It is unfair when a professional athlete loses a multimillion-dollar contract to someone whose size, strength, speed, or agility was enhanced illegally. Advocates of stricter enforcement of doping rules say that taking performance-enhancing drugs is no different than any other type of cheating and should be treated the same way as if a cyclist took the subway for part of the Tour de France or a professional athlete bribed an umpire or referee.

When some competitors are using drugs, others may see taking drugs themselves as the only way they can level the playing field. Some people believe that the best way to address the discrepancy between athletes who take performance-enhancing drugs and those who do not is to make performance enhancers legal. Allowing athletes to take the drugs legally would make the competition fairer, they say, because it would give everyone access to the same drugs. Taking performance-enhancing drugs would no longer be the best way to gain a competitive advantage. The drugs would simply become a routine part of an athlete's training regimen.

Advocates of legalizing performance-enhancing substances say this would make them safer. They point out that drugs have been used legally and illegally by athletes for many years, often under the care of professionals. "Insiders know that many—perhaps most—top players in all sports take drugs to train harder and feel no pain during play," says Adrianne Blue, a professor of journalism. "The trainers, sports doctors, nutritionists, physiotherapists and managers of the big names make sure banned substances are taken at the safest and most efficient levels."[36] If these drugs were legalized, there would be no reason to hide their use, increasing the information that trainers and users have at their disposal to ensure a safe dosage and identify warning signs of a problem.

Others argue that allowing all athletes to take drugs would be counterproductive because athletes would take more and more of the drug to retain their advantage. And given the potential damage to an athlete's health, linking success in sports to drugs would be immoral and unethical. Dr. Gary Gaffney, who writes a blog titled Steroid Nation, writes:

> If left unchecked, the use of doping to enhance performance will lead to a drug arms race (which has already happened) to see who can benefit most from drug use. Athletes will need multiple [performance-enhancing drugs]. Obviously these drugs will lead to significant morbidity and mortality.[37]

Do Performance-Enhancing Drugs Change the Outcome?

Athleticism depends on a wide range of physical, psychological, and lifestyle factors. In addition to innate ability, an athlete's skill level depends on his or her commitment and drive. An athlete's performance can be enhanced by the right trainer, coach, facility, and equipment. A strict training regimen, diet, and nutrition can further enhance performance. Given the many things that contribute to creating a winning athlete, some people believe that the impact of steroids has been overemphasized. Linda McMahon, the cofounder of World Wrestling Entertainment, says, "There is no competitive advantage for using steroids—it's not going to make you jump higher, run faster, hit the ball farther or anything like that."[38]

Many of the athletes who use steroids agree that the drugs are not miracle workers. For instance, Mark McGwire, who began using anabolic steroids to help him heal from an injury, contends that the drugs did not impact his performance. "I'm sure people will wonder if I could have hit all those home runs had I never taken steroids," he says. "I had good years when I didn't take any [steroids] and I had bad years when I didn't take any. I had good years when I took steroids and I had bad years when I took steroids."[39]

Athletes also contend that there is a fine line between the substances that are allowed and those that are not. Jennifer Sey, a U.S. national gymnast in the 1980s, writes that she "gobbled Advil like M&Ms" to overcome the daily pain of gymnastics competition and consumed "piles of laxatives in the herculean battle to keep my weight below 100 pounds, my body fat below 3 percent."[40] While neither ibuprofen nor laxatives are illegal, she sees no difference in the substances that have been banned: "I don't blame athletes like [U.S. sprinter] Marion Jones for juicing their performance with

U.S. Olympic swimmers model the LZR Racer swimsuits introduced by Speedo for the 2008 Beijing Olympics. The high-tech suits, which some critics called "performance enhancers," were later banned from international competitions.

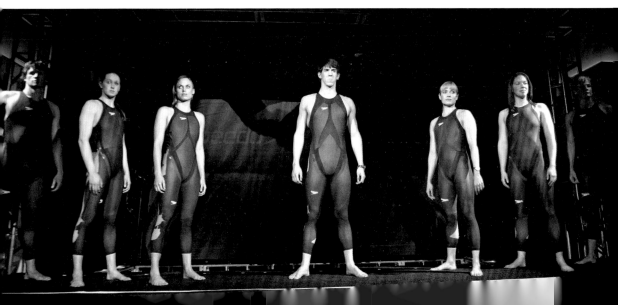

a little extra oomph. She's caught up in her sport; she needs that little somethin' . . . to maintain her edge."[41] Jones was stripped of the medals she won at the 1988 Olympic Games after she admitted using THG.

Most accomplished athletes achieve success without ever using drugs. Experts cite the fact that in the thousands of drug tests conducted prior to major sporting events, rarely do more than a handful of athletes test positive. Since testing was implemented at the Olympics, fewer and fewer athletes have been found to have used banned substances. At the 2010 Winter Games, only 1 athlete was disqualified due to a positive drug test. In addition, entire sports have been far removed from rumors of performance-enhancing drugs. Since the National Basketball Association began testing players for banned substances in 2001, just a handful of players have tested positive for steroids or other performance enhancers. And Major League Soccer handed out its first drug-related suspensions in 2009—9 years after the league began testing.

Technology Versus Athleticism

Some experts argue that performance-enhancing drugs are no different than other aspects of an athlete's training regimen. Athletes rely on all kinds of technical advances that improve performance; some experts believe that performance-enhancing substances should be viewed simply as another training tool. Gymnasts use springy pads that help them jump higher; skaters use new blades designed to help them go faster. A prime example is the high-tech LZR Racer swimsuit introduced by Speedo for the 2008 Olympics. This complex blend of high-tech materials is designed for maximum flotation and minimal resistance, a combination that one study found could take 1.9 to 2.2 percent off a swimmer's time in the 100-meter freestyle. In fact, 23 of the 25 swimmers who broke world records at the 2008 Summer Olympics, in which the LZR Racer made its debut, were wearing the swimsuit.

The International Swimming Federation, which governs international swimming events, had allowed the LZR Racer in 2008 and 2009 events, but the LZR was among the swimsuits that the International Swimming Federation later banned. The decision was based on the conclusion that the swimsuit provided an unfair advantage to the swimmers using it and undermined the spirit of fair play. In fact, some critics of the suit referred to it as a "performance enhancer."

Athletes also sometimes benefit from medical advances. Like other people with failing eyesight, athletes may use laser eye surgery

Major League Admissions

Throughout the first decade of the twenty-first century, headlines from newspapers and sports magazines screamed of the suspected use—and then the admitted use—of performance-enhancing drugs. Nowhere was this more common than Major League Baseball. After years of denial, many major league players admitted to using steroids. In 2010 Mark McGwire admitted to using anabolic steroids during his career and issued an apology. Alex Rodriguez also apologized for his use of the drugs. In 2009 he explained what led to his steroid use:

> When I arrived in Texas in 2001, I felt an enormous amount of pressure, felt all the weight of the world on top of me to perform and perform at a high level every day. Back then, it was a different culture. It was very loose. I was young, I was stupid, I was naive and I wanted to prove to everyone that I was worth, you know, being one of the greatest players of all time. And I did take a banned substance. For that, I'm very sorry and deeply regretful. And although it was the culture back then in Major League Baseball . . . I'm sorry for that time, I'm sorry to my fans, I'm sorry to my fans in Texas. It wasn't until then that I thought about substance of any kind, and since then I've proved to myself and to everyone that I don't need any of that.

Quoted in ESPN.com, "A-Rod Admits, Regrets Use of PEDs," interview with Peter Gammons, February 10, 2009. http://sports.espn.go.com.

(LASIK) to improve their eyesight. Following laser surgery, Tiger Woods's vision was improved to 20/15, meaning he can see at 20 yards (18.29m) what a person with "normal" eyesight would see at 15 yards (13.72m). Athletes often emerge stronger and more nimble following reconstructive surgery after an injury. In some cases a steroid or other drug is used to help an athlete return from injury more quickly. Whether a banned drug should be allowed to aid an athlete's recovery remains a topic of controversy.

The Impact on Fans

There is evidence that athletic organizations, coaches, and fans choose to overlook drug use by top athletes. In discussing football players and fans, Charles Yesalis, an expert on steroids and performance-enhancing drugs, argues that people "know these players are bigger, stronger and faster than the average Joe, but they want to see superheroes."[42]

Some fans may be willing to overlook drug use—and a lot of other negative behaviors—as long as they are entertained. Spectators want to see a winner. They love to watch records being broken. How these achievements are accomplished becomes of secondary importance. Sportswriter Philip Wolf is among those who say the use of drugs by athletes has no bearing on his enjoyment of the sport. "When Barry Bonds was mashing homers and his head looked like an enlarged potato, . . . fans like me didn't care. We just watch in fascination as the muscle-bound behemoth launched another 550-foot big fly."[43]

Still, many fans lament the use of drugs in athletics. In a survey taken in March 2005—in the aftermath of the BALCO scandal and in the midst of congressional hearings—40 percent of the baseball fans surveyed said that learning about steroid use in baseball had diminished their opinion of the game. In answer to the question, "Do fans really care about PEDs [performance-enhancing drugs]?" one blogger writes: "I care. I get mad at the players and all of baseball for letting it go on for so long. . . . I still cheer for the players I like [who have used performance-enhancing drugs], but sometimes not as loudly. And that makes me mad."[44]

"The illicit use of performance-enhancing substances—commonly referred to as 'doping'—is irreconcilable with the spirit of sport."[35]

— Paul C. McCaffrey, law associate.

44

For these fans, the thrill is in watching two or more equally matched competitors do everything they can to win—everything *within* the rules, however. Fans want to know that competitions are being determined by skill and athleticism, not by who can find the best combination of drugs. "I personally don't want to watch an event that is a pharmacology contest, with the winner being the person who can inject the most EPO without suffering cardiac arrest," writes a fan of the Tour de France. "All sports are fundamentally about testing the physical limits of humanity; drugs distort this test."[45]

The Impact on Sports' Image

Sports analysts worry about the impact that the media attention on performance-enhancing drugs has had on sports' image. Dr. Gary Gaffney, a professor of psychiatry at the University of Iowa College of Medicine, writes of the impact the steroid scandal in baseball could have on that sport's image: "If the MLB [Major League Baseball] wishes to maintain an image as a fair and regulated sport—a sport that protects the ethical integrity of the games and the health of the players—it will correct the PED [performance-enhancing drugs] problem."[46]

"There is no competitive advantage for using steroids—it's not going to make you jump higher, run faster, [or] hit the ball farther."[38]

— Linda McMahon, cofounder of World Wrestling Entertainment.

The use of performance-enhancing drugs undermines the ability of fans to relate to athletes and take pride in their accomplishments. Dr. Timothy Noakes writes, "Without the illusion that professional athletes are somewhat like ourselves, just better, their profession has no appeal. Rather, sport becomes no different from any other commercially driven activity."[47]

Each time an athlete is caught using a banned substance, it tarnishes the sport, its organizers, and athletes as a whole. By raising serious questions about many prominent athletes, the steroid scandals of the early years of the twenty-first century have made it more difficult for fans to embrace the accomplishments of their sports idols. "Fans no longer have the same connection with players and respect for the sport as a whole," says a writer about Major League Baseball. "They still root for their favorite team, but they may be less inclined to watch the Fox game of the week or a playoff series once their team is eliminated, because

PEDs [performance-enhancing drugs] have distanced players even more from the fans who adore them."[48]

Accusations and admissions of drug use have scandalized professional baseball since the late 1990s. While Americans expressed dismay about the prevalence of steroid use among ballplayers, some experts argue that there may be just as much drug use in other sports. Experts say that the NFL has ignored signs of anabolic steroid use among professional football players and warn of the possible repercussions. "Image counts for a great deal," writes Howard Bloom in an article in *Sports Business News*, "and when all is said and done the damage done to the NFL's image could hurt the economics of the game."[49]

Tarnished Reputations

Athletes who take performance-enhancing drugs also put their own reputation on the line. The steroid scandal that rocked Major League Baseball tarnished the reputations of a number of All-Star players. Those suspected of using performance-enhancing drugs were lambasted by the press, and their record-breaking achievements were called into question. Some say that such negative pub-

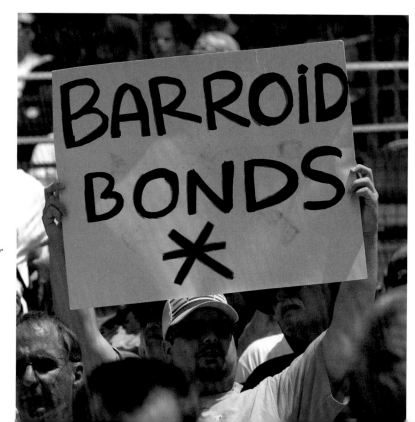

Home-run slugger Barry Bonds incurred the wrath of some fans, including this one, over allegations of steroid use. Bonds has denied using performance enhancers, but fans have grown weary of such denials—by Bonds and other athletes.

licity is the best deterrent for continued use. In a story on steroids in baseball, Josh Millar writes:

> Lift bans on performance enhancing drugs but KEEP the testing, make EVERY failed test in EVERY sport public knowledge. Let the players have their toughest fight—with themselves. Let the stars tarnish their own images and deal with their own mistakes. Let the court of public opinion decide. In a perfect world cheaters will be shunned and rule abiders praised.[50]

Some athletes caught taking illegal substances say they were unaware that they were taking a banned substance. Given the wide range of substances that are banned, honest mistakes might be expected. Sometimes athletes who are caught cheating blame their trainer. During the BALCO investigation, for instance, Barry Bonds admitted to receiving THG from his personal trainer, but Bonds said he thought that the drug was a treatment for arthritis. Marion Jones says her coach gave her THG for several months before she even knew what it was for. "He told me to put it under my tongue for a few seconds and swallow it," she said. "He told me not to tell anyone."[51] While skeptics dismiss such claims, athletes say they often follow the advice of their trainers without questioning the how or why of what they are doing.

Even under oath, athletes sometimes continue to deny their use of drugs. Jones vehemently denied doping allegations during the BALCO investigation. Her denial ruined her credibility and destroyed her career. When Jones admitted steroid use in 2007, the International Olympic Committee (IOC) stripped her of her medals and erased her records from the record books. Jones's drug use also impacted her teammates. In 2008 the IOC ruled that eight women involved in running relay races with Jones also had to return their medals. The women filed an appeal with the Court of Arbitration for Sport. "We are being unfairly punished," argued Chryste Gaines, who ran with Jones in the 2000 Olympic Games. "If the drug testing agencies cannot determine if an athlete is taking performance enhancing drugs how are the teammates supposed to know?"[52]

"I personally don't want to watch an event that is a pharmacology contest, with the winner being the person who can inject the most EPO without suffering cardiac arrest."[45]

— Jack Ewing, blogger and sports fan.

Study Shows hGH Helps Performance

In May 2010 researchers at the Garvan Institute of Medical Research in Sydney, Australia, reported findings supporting what performance-drug experts had long argued: that human growth hormone can boost athletic performance enough to make contests unfair between those who had taken the hormone and those who had not. The study tested the use of hGH in 103 male and female recreational athletes. For two months the athletes were injected with either hGH or salt water. Some of the male subjects also received testosterone. All subjects then lifted weights, jumped, and rode exercise bikes, while researchers compared their performance.

The improvement in performance with hGH was modest. In the study the hormone did not increase strength or endurance, but it did improve sprinting ability. Researchers say that athletes in running, swimming, or other events requiring a burst of energy would benefit most from hGH.

The research subjects who took hGH had a 4 percent increase in sprint capacity on a bicycle compared with the control population. Researchers estimate that this difference would amount to roughly half a second in a 100-meter race—enough time to separate the winner from the last-place finisher. When combined with testosterone, hGH had even greater impact, amounting to an 8 percent increase in sprinting ability.

The study used a smaller dose over a shorter period of time than athletes would probably use. Larger doses over a longer period of time could have an even greater impact on performance—and more dangerous side effects.

Lost Earnings

Many athletes also have a lot of money on the line. Marion Jones was making an estimated $3 million a year in endorsements and sponsorships when her admission of drug use ended her career. In some sports a suspension resulting from a positive test can cost an athlete hundreds of thousands of dollars. Los Angeles Dodger Manny Ramirez was suspended for 50 games after failing a drug test in May 2009. Ramirez lost an estimated $7.7 million in salary. Martina Hingis retired from tennis after a positive test for cocaine would have resulted in a two-year suspension. Hingis proclaimed her innocence but said that she had no interest in fighting the ban.

Early in 2010 a match between two of the world's top boxers, Floyd Mayweather Jr. and Manny Pacquiao, was canceled because they could not agree on drug-testing procedures after Mayweather accused Pacquiao of using performance-enhancing drugs. Sports analysts say that the fight could have been the highest-grossing boxing match in history. Each boxer would have earned an estimated $25 million.

The Cloud of Suspicion

The more often athletes are caught using banned substances or admit to their use in the past, the more others are under suspicion. Each time a record is broken, fans wonder whether the athlete was under the influence of performance-enhancing drugs. The most cynical among the fans may assume that everyone is doping. Wolf writes, "When Ben Johnson crossed that finish line in 9.79 seconds during the 1988 Summer Olympics, I didn't care what was in his body because I figured every one of his competitors was doing the same thing."[53]

Some experts defend the athletes who use performance-enhancing drugs. Driven by their desire to win and the pressure to succeed, they say, the temptation to use a performance-enhancing drug can be staggering. All great athletes want to win, and they make many sacrifices to achieve this goal. In Major League Baseball the difference between a good batting average and a great one can mean millions of dollars. Moreover, athletes may be persuaded by a coach, trainer, teammate, or other trusted advisor to take a performance enhancer. Athletes need protection from the temptation to give in to these outside influences. Some sports enthusiasts say that strict guidelines and strong enforcement measures are needed to keep performance-enhancing drug use in check.

"When Ben Johnson crossed that finish line in 9.79 seconds during the 1988 Summer Olympics, I didn't care what was in his body because I figured every one of his competitors was doing the same thing."[53]

— Philip Wolf, deputy editor and columnist, *Ottawa Citizen*.

FACTS

- A 2007 study of Major League Baseball players undertaken by Emory University concluded that offensive production increased approximately 12 percent in steroid users versus nonusers.

- A 2008 *New York Times*/CBS News poll found that 53 percent of baseball fans said that it mattered a lot to them whether a player used steroids. Twenty-nine percent said it mattered a little, and 16 percent said it did not matter at all.

- In a 2006 survey, 82 percent of baseball fans said the use of steroids among players called into question several baseball records.

- In a 2008 survey of 1,000 student-athletes in elite athletic programs, over 92 percent said that using steroids was "cheating."

- In a 2008 survey, 20 percent of high school students said that anabolic steroid use by professional athletes influenced their own decision to use steroids. When students were asked whether athletes' use of steroids influenced their friends' decisions to use anabolic steroids, nearly 50 percent said yes.

- In a 2008 Gallup poll, 35 percent of respondents said that they suspected performance-enhancing drugs were involved when track-and-field athletes break records, and 22 percent suspect drug use when swimmers set new records.

- In a 2008 *New York Times*/CBS News poll, 34 percent of the fans estimated that at least half of Major League Baseball players used steroids or other performance-enhancing drugs; 36 percent said about a quarter of the players did, and 22 percent said only a few players used the drugs.

Should Sports Organizations Take Stronger Measures to Stop Performance-Enhancing Drugs?

Almost all national and international sports governing organizations have policies outlawing the use of performance enhancers. Many athletic organizations follow the guidelines and the list of banned substances developed by WADA. WADA includes a substance on the World Anti-Doping Code Prohibited List if it meets two of the following three criteria: (1) it is performance-enhancing, (2) it is harmful to the athlete's health, and (3) it violates the spirit of sport. WADA bans substances such as anabolic agents, hormones, diuretics, and stimulants, as well as methods such as blood transfusions and gene manipulation. As of December 2009 WADA's list included 192 substances and methods.

There is evidence that setting strict guidelines and aggressively pursuing cheaters can have an effect on the use of performance

State High School Screening Programs

Four states have established steroid screening programs at the high school level. In 2006 New Jersey became the first state to establish a program. New Jersey's program applies only to athletes who belong to teams in statewide tournaments. Athletes who test positive are banned from competition for one year. Illinois's program, which was established by the Illinois High School Association, began in 2008. The program conducts random testing of athletes competing in sectional, regional, and championship games.

The programs in Florida and Texas were established by an action of the state legislature. Before it was dropped in 2009, Florida's program included random testing of 1 percent of athletes on high school weight-lifting, football, and baseball teams. A student with a positive result received a 90-day suspension. Texas's program is the most far-reaching of the state programs. It covers more than 40,000 athletes in all sports and includes random testing of 3 percent of these athletes. Texas uses a tiered approach to penalties. The first positive result receives a 30-day suspension and the second a 1-year suspension. If an athlete tests positive 3 times, he or she is permanently banned from competition.

enhancers among athletes. Some people believe that the reason steroid scandals have rocked Major League Baseball and not the NFL is because the NFL has clearer policies regarding the use of performance enhancers and implements stronger enforcement mechanisms. The NFL was the first U.S. professional sports league to crack down on steroid use; it began to suspend players in 1989—more than a decade before Major League Baseball began its ban. Sports governing organizations for younger athletes—those in college and high school—also have enacted rigorous rules to prevent the use of performance-enhancing drugs from becoming a part of competition at these levels.

Testing for Drug Use in High Schools

Studies of the National Institute on Drug Abuse and the Centers for Disease Control and Prevention show a declining use of steroids and other performance-enhancing drugs among high school students. Still, experts warn that any use among young people is a topic of concern, and that the use of illegal substances among some at-risk groups may be as high as 6 to 12 percent. The use of steroids among young football players is an area of particular concern. Repeated studies show that high school football players are heavier than ever; experts say this is an indication that steroids, creatine, and other performance enhancers are prevalent. In some schools the use of these substances is also increasing in other sports, including baseball, tennis, and cheerleading.

In 2006 New Jersey became the first state to require random drug testing for high school athletes. New Jersey contracts with the National Center for Drug Free Sport to conduct random tests on athletes who qualify for state championships. The tests target sports in which there may be a high risk of doping, such as football, wrestling, and track and field. Of the 500 students tested in the first year, just one tested positive.

Since New Jersey's law, at least three other states— Florida, Texas, and Illinois—have passed legislation mandating random testing of high school athletes. These programs require all athletes in high school sports to be tested at random; athletes who test positive or refuse to be tested can be suspended from competition.

> *"[Drug] testing is deterring our young people from putting their lives at risk or wrecking their bodies through the use of illegal steroids."* [54]
>
> — Texas lieutenant governor David Dewhurst.

Outside of the states in which testing is mandated, few schools have aggressive programs that test athletes for performance-enhancing drugs. According to the National Institute on Drug Abuse, only about 9 percent of secondary schools conduct any type of drug testing program for athletes, and less than 4 percent of the nation's high schools test athletes for steroids. One of the obstacles is the cost. The average cost for a test for steroids is $104, which many schools simply cannot afford.

Limitations of Drug Testing in High School

Studies are under way to determine whether testing reduces drug abuse. Early tests have had few positive results. Of the first 10,000 students tested under Texas's new law, just 4 tested positive (22 refused to take the test). New Jersey tested 500 state championship athletes in 2006, and only 1 of the students had a positive test. Advocates of mandatory drug-testing programs take this as proof that the drug tests are working. "[Drug] testing is deterring our young people from putting their lives at risk or wrecking their bodies through the use of illegal steroids,"[54] says Texas lieutenant governor David Dewhurst.

The biggest obstacle to drug testing in schools is the sheer number of student-athletes. "The problem with testing is that it's hard to know who to test. You have all these young people from recreational school athletes, to college athletes, down to Little League,"[55] says Dr. Edward V. Craig, a sports medicine specialist at the Hospital for Special Surgery in New York. When to conduct tests is another issue. Craig adds: "Some states have tried [testing] prior to tournaments, but if athletes know when they're going to be tested, they can stop using the drugs. It's hugely expensive to have a state try to test every high school athlete."[56]

Drug abuse experts warn that high school drug-testing programs focus on team sports rather than individual sports. Some also may fail to address the growing use of steroids among high school students who take the drugs to look good rather than to improve athletic performance. Experts warn that girls may be at particular risk of being overlooked by drug-prevention programs. In 2008 Dionne Roberts went public with her experiences with anabolic steroids. In 2003 Roberts, a cheerleader, gymnast, and student body vice president of her Texas high school, said she bought anabolic steroids from a friend on the football team. "I was the last person in the world you'd think would use anabolic steroids,"[57] she says. Like many other girls, she used the drugs for cosmetic reasons. It is no longer enough for a woman to be thin; the ideal female body is lean yet muscular—a look that girls believe can be achieved through using steroids. "It's not uncommon to strive for that four-pack or six-pack, even in girls," says Roberts. "Being in shape is not just a masculine thing."[58] Roberts wound up with depression and attempted suicide before deciding to use her experience to warn others of the dangers of steroids.

Some people believe that the money could be better spent on other prevention efforts. "The vast majority of high schoolers are never going to touch steroids during their athletic career," writes George Spellwin, who runs an Internet site for bodybuilders. "The ones who do juice are so few that it makes testing seem worthless. And when you factor in how many millions of dollars get put towards testing then you're just talking about a huge waste of taxpayer money."[59] Several legislators have sought to reverse the state laws. In fact, Florida dropped its state-funded random drug-testing program in February 2009, citing a lack of money.

High school athletes in Chicago sign a pledge to not use steroids. The "I Play Clean" pledge-signing event is part of a campaign by NFL Hall of Famer Dick Butkus to teach young athletes the risks of steroid use.

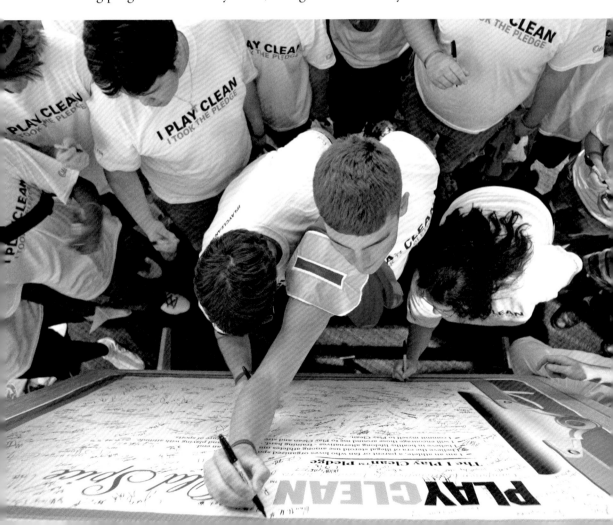

NCAA Programs

The National Collegiate Athletic Association (NCAA) has spear-headed education efforts for more than 30 years to deter the use of performance enhancers by college athletes. The NCAA began testing athletes involved in championships and postseason football in 1986. Since then it has expanded the breadth of its drug-testing policy.

Today the NCAA's list of banned drug classes is far more extensive than those substances banned under federal law. The NCAA tests athletes for the use of steroids, masking agents, and ephedrine, as well as other stimulants, hormones, and street drugs.

The NCAA spends approximately $4 million each year for its national drug-testing program. The NCAA has the National Center for Drug Free Sport test all divisions of its athletes at team and individual championships. At all rounds of NCAA championship events, athletes can be selected randomly for testing or chosen based on position, playing time, or place of finish. Athletes at Division I and II schools may also be subject to off-season testing.

On average, roughly 1 percent of the athletes tested under the NCAA program have tested positive for a banned substance. The general trend is toward fewer positive results. While program sponsors say this is evidence that the program is working, others suggest that the decline may be because athletes have figured out how to dupe the test. Some critics of the NCAA program also argue that many of the students who test positive do not realize they are doing anything wrong. "Most college students who report a positive drug test are because of substances, including steroids, found in over-the-counter supplements,"[60] says Dr. Gary Green, chair of the NCAA drug-testing committee.

Sanctions from a positive drug test are automatic. After the first positive test, a student-athlete cannot compete in any intercollegiate sport for one year; a second positive test results in the student being banned from intercollegiate competition. The NCAA bans also apply to any athlete suspended by a sports governing body that has adopted the WADA code.

Anti-Doping Policies of Professional Athletic Organizations

Each professional sports league is responsible for creating and enforcing its own anti-doping regulations. A brief description of the anti-doping measures undertaken in a few popular sports follows.

Tennis: The International Tennis Federation, which oversees the program for professional tennis players, tests players during events and conducts unscheduled tests between competitions. The federation typically tests semifinalists at each tournament and also has the discretion to target players who are suspected of drug use. One positive test results in disqualification and a two-year suspension; a second failed test results in a lifelong ban.

Golf: Both the Professional Golf Association and the Ladies Professional Golf Association began their first performance-enhancing drug testing programs in 2008. Both organizations conduct random and targeted testing at tournaments, with no minimum or maximum number of tests per year. The list of performance-enhancing drugs includes beta blockers, because of their ability to diminish the effect of adrenaline and steady a player's swing, and marijuana, due to its perceived calming effect. The Professional Golf Association's policy also allows random tests to be conducted apart from competitions and includes a provision that would allow doping allegations to be brought against players suspected of drug use in the past.

Boxing: Boxing is regulated by the gaming commission in each state in which matches are held. Most states test for steroids in some capacity. In 2002 the New York State Athletic Commission became the first to implement mandatory steroid testing before each fight. In January 2008 Nevada introduced random, unannounced tests on licensed fighters throughout the year.

College Drug-Testing Programs

About half of U.S. colleges and universities have their own drug-testing programs in place. These programs test for recreational drugs, such as marijuana and cocaine, far more often than for performance enhancers, however. Just 12 percent of the samples collected in 2007 were tested for anabolic steroids. In addition, testing is far more prevalent in schools with strong athletic programs than in other schools. In 2007 just 18 percent of Division III schools—smaller colleges with less emphasis on sports—had drug-testing programs in place.

Antidrug advocates argue that testing should be required of all colleges, regardless of their size, quality of athletic programs, and level of competition. Students at smaller schools may be just as likely to use steroids or other performance enhancers to make the team, they say. Athletes at colleges without drug testing might be more tempted to take banned substances. This not only raises issues about the fairness of intercollegiate competitions but also increases the risk that athletes will be tempted to dope to even out the playing field.

The Olympics and Amateur Sports

The IOC's rules are based on WADA's regulations, but they are more restrictive. According to the rules, athletes caught using a banned substance are banned from competition. The IOC also can disqualify the entire team if more than one member is found to have committed an anti-doping rule violation. In weight lifting, for instance, in which the use of anabolic steroids has been particularly problematic, the IOC instituted a "3 strikes" rule: If three of a country's team members test positive for steroid use in a year, the country's entire Olympic weight-lifting team is disqualified from competition. The policy resulted in weight-lifting teams from Romania and Bulgaria being banned from the 2000 Olympics.

The IOC believes that doping at the Olympics is less widespread than it was in the 1980s and 1990s. In part this is because far fewer national governments and Olympic teams encourage athletes to take anabolic steroids or other performance-enhancing drugs. In fact, many countries have formed their own drug-testing and enforcement organizations, based on the WADA code. In the United States all Olympic athletes are under the jurisdiction of the U.S. Anti-Doping Agency (USADA), which follows WADA's code. The USADA reserves the right to conduct unannounced tests on Olympic athletes in any sport at any time, year-round. The athlete's ranking, drug-test history, and the sport's risk of doping are taken into account when determining the testing strategy.

Advances in testing capabilities also have contributed to the decline. Whereas athletes once were tested at the Olympic Games themselves—often after they had participated in their event—the IOC today oversees an expansive program to test Olympic athletes prior to the games. In 2010 at least 30 athletes were caught violating doping rules long before the Winter Olympics began and were barred from competition. Of the 2,100 drug tests conducted during the games, just one athlete was suspended: Polish cross-country skier Kornelia Marek was disqualified after testing positive for EPO. There were also two minor violations—both involving hockey players who tested positive for light stimulants and were let off with reprimands.

The IOC believes the results show that its drug bans and enforcement methods are working. Dr. Arne Lundqvist, chair of the IOC's medical commission, called "the relative absence of doping" at the 2010 Olympic Games "a very encouraging message. It really tells us that efforts by national federations and world anti-doping agencies is more and more efficient."[61]

"If you are caught [taking performance-enhancing drugs], you should be banned forever. That would be a deterrent."[65]

— Chris Chelios, American professional ice hockey player.

One challenge that remains is keeping up with the ever-changing drugs. In some cases athletes are caught only after they have been using a banned substance for many years. To counter such criticisms, in 2010 the IOC initiated a policy to retain doping samples for 8 years to enable them to be reanalyzed based on new tests for drugs that the IOC has not yet identified. The IOC also plans to improve on its current methods by collecting "biological passports" for Olympic athletes. Biological passports provide baseline readings describing an athlete's red blood cell count and urine protein profile. A significant change in these levels could be used as an indication of doping. Prior to the 2010 Winter Olympics, the IOC issued a two-year suspension to German speed skater Claudia Pechstein because her blood tests showed abnormally high levels of red blood cells compared with her baseline test.

Professional Sports

Several international sports organizations, including the International Tennis Federation and the Fédération Internationale de Football Association, follow many of the guidelines put forth by WADA. Major League Baseball, the NFL, the National Basketball Association (NBA), the Women's National Basketball Association (WNBA), and the National Hockey League (NHL) are among the organizations that have chosen to develop their own list of banned substances rather than adopt WADA's code.

Although all major U.S. sports leagues have some type of program in place, they often have less-aggressive testing policies than WADA. For instance, neither the NBA, the WNBA, nor the NHL requires players to be tested annually; each of these organizations also has a cap on the number of times a player can be tested in any year. Professional leagues also often ban far fewer substances than WADA and have less-aggressive penalties for cheating. The NFL's list of banned substances, for instance, includes just 10 stimulants; WADA's list includes 50. The NFL's four-day suspension for first-time violators does not compare with WADA's two-year suspension.

One reason for the discrepancy between the way doping is handled at the professional and amateur levels might have to do with the amount of money involved. When a star player is suspended, fewer people may attend games. In professional sports a suspension that lasts two or more years could have a profound effect on revenues for the team and the league as a whole. Drug scandals may also result in a loss of sponsors. Several corporations, including the Discovery Channel, Audi, and Adidas, ended their long-term sponsorship of Tour de France teams in the wake of doping allegations. In 2007, Deutsche Telekom, the main sponsor of the T-Mobile team, cited doping as

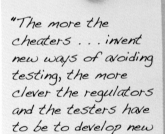

"The more the cheaters . . . invent new ways of avoiding testing, the more clever the regulators and the testers have to be to develop new tests."[66]

— Theodore Friedmann, head of the World Anti-Doping Agency's gene doping panel.

one of the main reasons it ended its involvement with the Tour after 16 years. In some sports, athletes are dependent on sponsors to pay their salaries and expenses; in others, elite athletes may earn far more from endorsements and sponsorships than from their salary or winnings. "In the present climate, the hint of a drugs connection is enough to switch off the money tap," writes John Humphrys, a television host for the British Broadcasting Corporation. "Sponsors back away from tainted athletes as swiftly as they cosy up to them when they are winning the medals. The television companies, who also pump millions into the sport, might take fright, too. The money might disappear." [62]

Enforcing the Rules

Even with random drug tests, some people doubt whether sports organizations are truly interested in catching cheaters. Some professional leagues have been criticized for having lax testing protocols and enforcement mechanisms. Gary Wadler, an expert on drug use in sports, says that most organizations for professional athletes address drug use only when the media and fans force their hand. "I think most people in professional sports wish the problem away," he says. "They tweak their programs to take the heat off."[63]

Major League Baseball is a case in point. It had few penalties in place until the media began to focus attention on the rampant use of steroids among major league players. In 2006 the league began a "three strikes and you're out" policy. Under this proposal, a player receives a 50-game suspension for a first positive test, 100 games for the second, and a lifetime ban for the third.

The NHL's performance-enhancing drug policy is full of loopholes. Under the policy in place in 2010, the NHL can test teams without notice up to three times a year, but in fact teams are tested less frequently. In addition, the NHL does not test for steroids or other drugs during the playoffs. Experts say such policies do not go far enough. "You would have to be an idiot to get caught under a system like that—an absolute moron," said Charles Yesalis, a Penn State University professor who specializes in the use and impact of performance-enhancing substances. "To me, you have to go far beyond that testing system to have a true sense of whether players [are or] are not doping."[64] In fact, since the policy went into effect, only one player has tested positive for a banned substance.

According to the NHL's policy, a player caught cheating is suspended the first two times but banned from play if caught a third time. After two years, however, a banned player can request to be reinstated. NHL legend Chris Chelios says the penalties are not strong enough. "If you are caught, you should be banned forever. That would be a deterrent," he says. "I'm willing to take it a step further and start blood-testing athletes."[65]

Chelios is not alone in his criticism that the NHL has not done enough to eliminate drug use among professional hockey players. In 2008 Columbus Blue Jacket Bryan Berard tested positive for anabolic steroids as part of the testing to be considered for the U.S. Olympic hockey team. Berard was banned from international competition for two years, but because the test was not administered by the NHL, the NHL allowed him to continue to play—a policy that WADA president Dick Pound described as seriously flawed.

Drug Testing as a Deterrent

Experts disagree on the effectiveness of random drug testing as a deterrent. Some people say that a low percentage of positive drug tests suggests that the greater the risk of getting caught, the less likely an athlete will be to take a banned substance. Others say that a low percentage of positive tests is an indication that athletes have figured out how to beat the system. With some drugs, athletes can time the dosage so that the drug is out of their system before providing a urine sample for testing. Some athletes have used more extreme measures, such as using a catheter to fill their bladder with drug-free urine before a test or pouring alcohol into the urine sample to mask an illegal drug.

One of the problems with enforcing bans is that it is simply impossible to test every athlete for every potential performance-enhancing drug. This is particularly problematic given the ever-changing nature of the drugs. "It's . . . a constant tug of war between the cheaters and the regulators," says Theodore Friedmann. "And the more the cheaters kind of modify their methods and invent new ways of avoiding testing, the more clever the regulators and the testers have to be to develop new tests."[66]

The establishment of WADA has led to better coordination of drug testing and punishment throughout the international sports community. WADA's research branch is charged with tracking new drugs and developing tests before they reach widespread use. As a result, tests are being added each year, and administrators say the tests are becoming increasingly reliable in detecting new forms of doping. In February 2010 British rugby player Terry Newton became the first athlete to test positive for overly high levels of hGH—a banned performance-enhancing substance whose use has been difficult to detect because it occurs naturally in the body.

While some organizations have taken strong measures to curb the use of performance-enhancing drugs in and beyond athletics, others have a long way to go. Experts warn that, given the amount of money to be made by professional athletes and the organizations for which they work, many athletic organizations are under pressure to look the other way when a star athlete is suspected of drug use. Sports organizers may be unable to stamp out drug use on their own; prevention will likely require stronger law enforcement to curb supply and educational programs aimed at reducing demand.

Urine samples await testing for drugs at the Olympic Analytical Laboratory at the University of California at Los Angeles. Some athletes have found ways to mask use of banned performance-enhancing substances.

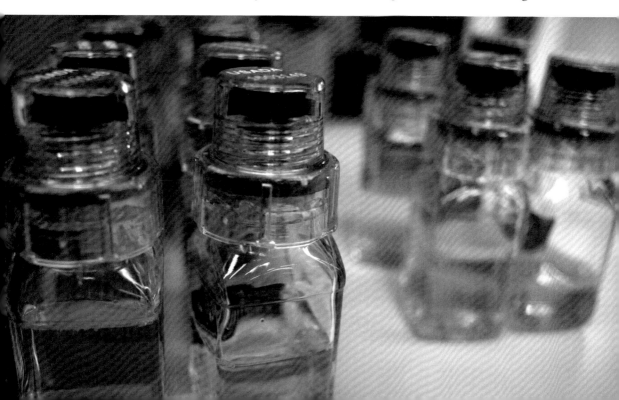

FACTS

- The International Olympic Committee began testing athletes for drugs in 1968 and has tested athletes ever since, adding tests for new performance-enhancing drugs as they become available.

- The World Anti-Doping Agency has banned 192 performance-enhancing substances and methods (as of December 22, 2008), including alcohol, marijuana, testosterone, insulin, blood transfusions, and gene manipulation.

- As of December 2008, 625 sports organizations worldwide had adopted the World Anti-Doping Agency's code banning 192 performance-enhancing substances and methods.

- The U.S. Anti-Doping Agency reports that fewer than 1 percent of the 8,532 athlete drug tests conducted in 2008 (the most recent year available) identified potential doping violations.

- A 2008 Gallup poll showed that fans are divided as to whether the International Olympic Committee is doing enough to deal with the use of performance-enhancing drugs by Olympic athletes, with 50 percent saying it is doing enough and 44 percent saying it is not.

- Random steroid tests cost roughly $104 each, compared with an average of $18 for tests for recreational drugs.

- The National Hockey League policy calls for a player who tests positive for a banned substance to be suspended for 20 games for the first offense, suspended for 60 games for the second offense, and banned for life for the third offense.

- Fifty-nine cases of doping violations resulted from the 21,579 drug tests conducted at the Summer Olympics between 1968 and 2008. There have been 14 positive results from 7,364 tests conducted at the Winter Olympics between 1968 and 2010.

CHAPTER FIVE

How Can the Use of Performance- Enhancing Drugs Be Prevented?

Experts warn that as long as there is demand for performance-enhancing drugs, the use of these drugs will continue. At any level of competition, the incentives for excelling in sports may outweigh the risk of getting caught. For a high school student, a college scholarship may be in the balance; an Olympic or professional athlete may feel that getting a spot on the team depends on doing everything possible.

Steroids, stimulants, and other drugs are relatively easy to obtain. Antidrug advocates believe that prevention can succeed only by addressing supply as well as demand. This would require stepping up law enforcement strategies to eliminate the smuggling of drugs into the country, the manufacture of drugs in clandestine labs, and the sale of drugs over the Internet.

Critics say current laws have done little to curb the use of performance-enhancing drugs among some segments of the population. Even as major drug busts have led to the arrest of suppliers, anabolic steroids, EPOs, and other drugs remain readily available. Antidrug advocates say that a multipronged approach is needed to address performance-enhancing drug use. Success will depend on combining stringent law enforcement efforts targeted at both supply and demand with educational programs for athletes of all levels. Ensuring that the risks of using these drugs are greater than the benefits will be the key to success.

Laws Governing the Use of Performance-Enhancing Drugs

There were few regulations regarding some of the most common performance-enhancing drugs prior to the 1960s, when their short- and long-term health risks first became evident. Since then the United States has enacted many laws intended to reduce both the demand and supply of performance-enhancing drugs. The use of anabolic steroids and other drugs for the purpose of enhancing athletic performance is not only against the rules of competition, it is also illegal.

The Controlled Substances Act of 1970 is the primary U.S. law governing illegal drugs. The act includes 5 schedules—or categories—of drugs. Drugs are categorized primarily based on their medical uses, likelihood of abuse, and health risks. Heroin, for instance, is classified as a Schedule I drug because it has no medical uses and is highly addictive. At the other end of the spectrum are Schedule V drugs: those that are widely prescribed to treat common ailments and do not have a high risk of abuse. Schedule V drugs include cough syrups with codeine and mild painkillers. The Anabolic Steroid Control Act of 1990 classified anabolic steroids as Schedule III drugs. Possessing a Schedule III drug without a prescription is a federal crime, punishable by up to one year in prison, a minimum fine of $1,000, or both. The illegal sale of steroids carries a punishment of up to 10 years in prison and a $250,000 fine. In 2004 Congress expanded the list of illegal drugs to include precursors to steroids—which are substances that can be converted by the body into anabolic steroids—as well as the raw materials used to manufacture synthetic steroids.

Since then Congress has continued to hold hearings to address the continuing problem. In the wake of the scandal that rocked Major League Baseball during the first decade of the 2000s, for instance, Congress held a series of hearings into the use

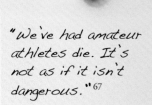

"We've had amateur athletes die. It's not as if it isn't dangerous."[67]

— John McCain, U.S. senator and advocate for strong performance-enhancement drug legislation.

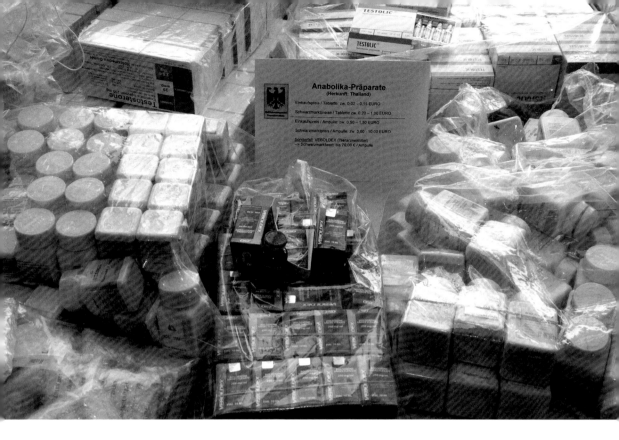

Steroids seized by German authorities are displayed for the news media in 2009. Performance-enhancing drugs are illegal in many nations. In the United States, possession of anabolic steroids without a prescription is a federal crime.

of performance-enhancing drugs in sports. Congress has considered legislation that would mandate a universal anti-doping policy for every U.S. professional sports league, but no action has yet been taken. Dietary supplements have also been the target of lawmakers. Senator John McCain introduced legislation on February 3, 2010, that would require manufacturers of dietary supplements to register with the FDA and to disclose the ingredients used in their products. McCain said the Dietary Supplement Safety Act is intended to protect athletes at any level who use supplements to boost their performance. "We've had amateur athletes die," said McCain in an interview. "It's not as if it isn't dangerous."[67]

McCain believes his bill not only would help to protect people from unsafe supplements, it also would help athletes know whether or not a supplement had any banned ingredients. Several athletes who have tested positive under various drug programs have blamed unlabeled substances in dietary supplements. In explaining why he introduced the legislation, McCain said that a "little over a year ago the NFL suspended six players . . . for violating the

Challenges to Mandatory Drug-Testing Policies

The American Civil Liberties Union is among the organizations that have challenged the right of schools to conduct mandatory drug tests for students. Lawyers argue that mandatory testing is a violation of a student's right to privacy. They further argue that drug testing is only constitutional when there is a reason for suspicion. Some people say that "suspicionless" drug testing of high school students engaged in extracurricular activities is aimed at the students least likely to get in trouble with drugs and will scare away youth at risk of drug use from participating in after-school programs, which have been proven to be effective drug-prevention tools.

The Supreme Court has ruled on this issue several times. In the 1995 case *Vernonia School District v. Acton*, the Court upheld an Oregon's school's policy to conduct drug testing of student-athletes. In a 2002 case the Court overruled an appeals court that had decided Tecumseh, Oklahoma, Public School District's drug-testing policy was unconstitutional. The policy required high school students participating in any extracurricular activities—academic, artistic, and so on—to submit to drug tests. The federal court had ruled this policy to be unconstitutional because there was no suspicion that any of the students tested had ever used illegal drugs or that the school had a widespread drug problem.

league's anti-doping policy. Several of the players were surprised that they tested positive for a banned substance because they used a dietary supplement they believed to be safe and legal."[68]

Law Enforcement

The Drug Enforcement Administration (DEA) is responsible for enforcing federal laws related to illegal drug use, including those used to enhance performance. Part of the DEA's enforcement mechanisms include uncovering performance-enhancing drugs as they are smuggled into the United States, locating laboratories that illegally manufacture these drugs, and identifying pharmacies that illegally distribute them. Several of the DEA's investigations have been undertaken in conjunction with the U.S. Anti-Doping Agency and other sports governing organizations, as well as local law enforcement agencies. Since 2000 the DEA and other law enforcement agencies have become increasingly focused on anabolic steroids, leading to the arrest and indictment of hundreds of doctors, pharmacists, and users.

Most of the illegal steroids in the United States are smuggled into the country from Mexico and European countries in which a prescription is not required for the purchase of steroids. Some other performance-enhancing drugs are diverted from legitimate sources through theft or prescription forgery, and some are manufactured in unlawful laboratories.

The most publicized federal investigation into performance-enhancing drugs took place in 2002, when DEA agents raided the Bay Area Laboratory Co-Operative (BALCO), a laboratory that had been illegally manufacturing THG. Documents found at the lab cast suspicion of illegal steroid use on a number of well-known athletes, including Major League Baseball stars Jason Giambi and Barry Bonds, U.S. sprinter Marion Jones, and NFL Super Bowl champion Bill Romanowski. More than 30 elite athletes testified before a grand jury, broadening media coverage of the incident. Four men—BALCO founder Victor Conte, BALCO executive James Valente, track coach Remi Korchemny, and trainer Greg Anderson (who worked with Barry Bonds, among others)—were indicted on 42 counts, including conspiracy to distribute anabolic steroids. In 2005 Conte and Anderson pleaded guilty to steroid distribution and money laundering. Conte received a sentence of 4 months in prison and 4 months under house arrest; Anderson was sentenced to 3 months in prison and 3 months under house arrest. Valente and Korchemny were each given a 1-year probation. Several athletes were convicted of perjury—lying under oath—when testifying before the grand jury.

"It is common knowledge that steroids are readily available in gymnasiums and health clubs."[71]

— Bruce Svare, director of the National Institute for Sports Reform.

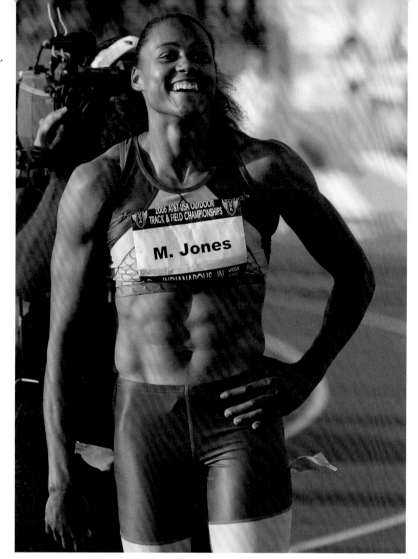

Sprinter Marion Jones celebrates her win in the women's 100-meter dash at the 2006 U.S. Outdoor Track & Field Championships. Jones was one of many prominent athletes named in documents seized from a lab that illegally manufactured steroids.

Cracking Down

The largest federal crackdown on illegal steroids happened in September 2007, in a DEA sting called Operation Raw Deal. The DEA hit every aspect of the underground network, from manufacturing to distribution to the actual buyers. The DEA found 56 laboratories that were being used to manufacture steroids illegally, seized 533 pounds (242kg) of raw steroid powder, and arrested 124 people. According to the charges, the dealers purchased the powder on the Internet and received directions on how to convert it into useable drugs. In the international investigation, the DEA worked with drug agents from Mexico, Germany, Denmark, and Thailand.

To meet the demand for performance-enhancing drugs, a growing number of interstate and international distribution chains are emerging, mirroring the supply chains of other illegal drugs. While some people believe that anabolic steroids are safe, the conditions exposed by Operation Raw Deal suggest otherwise. The steroid powder, which originally came from China, was being manufactured in unsanitary kitchens and garages by people who knew little or nothing about chemistry.

The government has also targeted the illegal sale of steroids and other performance-enhancing drugs via Internet sites. Experts say that some of the drugs for sale over the Internet may be smuggled in from other countries, but often they are made illegally in unsanitary kitchen and basement labs. To counter this problem, in 2006 the FBI initiated Operation Phony Pharm, which targets Web sites and individuals illegally selling steroids and hGH over the Internet. "The dangers associated with the improper use of steroids and human growth hormone are well documented," said Kevin J. O'Connor, U.S. Attorney for the District of Connecticut. "However, this investigation has helped to shed light on additional troubling concerns, including the manufacture of these drugs in unsanitary kitchen and basement labs, and their subsequent sale on web sites, many of which are frequented by minors." [69]

"I'm the one who decided to lie about using performance-enhancing drugs. I am the one who decided to lie to myself because I was trying to avoid certain consequences." [75]

— Marion Jones, track and field athlete who was stripped of her Olympic medals after admitting to steroid use.

Oversight of Dietary Supplements Increases

The FDA also has played a role in addressing performance-enhancing drugs by stepping up oversight of dietary supplements. In 2009, for instance, the FDA sent a warning to American Cellular Labs, which was positioning eight anabolic steroid products as dietary supplements on its Web site. Margaret Hamburg, the commissioner of the FDA, explains the need for stringent enforcement:

The site promotes the products with claims like, "MASS Xtreme is perfect if you are focused on adding muscle mass, power and strength to your physique," and "ESTRO Xtreme . . . you get two estrogen blocking effects in one fantastic product!"

In fact, these over-the-counter body-building products have been associated with serious and life-threatening adverse effects, including liver injury, stroke, kidney failure, and pulmonary embolism.[70]

Strategies to curb availability are important aspects of the solution to any illegal drug problem, but law enforcement is not enough. Bruce Svare, a professor at the University of Albany and director of the National Institute for Sports, writes:

> It is common knowledge that steroids are readily available in gymnasiums and health clubs. The recent uncovering of clandestine pharmacies and underground laboratories as well as offshore Internet Web sites (the federal Drug Enforcement [Administration] estimates 4,000 transactions a day), is not surprising to those of us who have studied the problem. Unfortunately, for every illicit laboratory, pharmacy and Web site detected and prosecuted, hundreds, probably thousands, more operate with little interference.[71]

Prevention Through Education

A number of public and private organizations are involved in antidrug campaigns intended to educate Americans about the dangers of performance-enhancing drugs. The Partnership for a Drug-Free America, which focuses on education and awareness programs intended to prevent young people from using drugs, provides information on steroids and several other drugs sometimes used to enhance performance. The organization has produced several TV spots on the dangers of performance-enhancing drugs. In one, launched during the 2005 Major League Baseball All-Star Game, the statue of an athlete crumbles to represent how steroids destroy a young person's body, as the voice-over shares some of the risks to young athletes.

A number of federal government agencies also have targeted performance-enhancing drugs in their drug-prevention activities. The National Institute on Drug Abuse and the White House Office of National Drug Control Policy include education

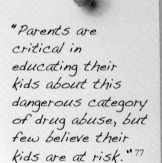

"Parents are critical in educating their kids about this dangerous category of drug abuse, but few believe their kids are at risk."[77]

— Steve Pasierb, president and CEO of the Partnership for a Drug-Free America.

ATLAS and ATHENA

ATLAS (Athletes Training and Learning to Avoid Steroids) and ATHENA (Athletes Targeting Healthy Exercise and Nutrition Alternatives) are award-winning, evidence-based health promotion and substance abuse–prevention programs for high school athletic teams.

ATLAS and ATHENA educate athletes about sports nutrition, strength training, and the effects of drugs on performance. The peer-led approach is part of what makes the programs effective. Student-athletes teach each other in a small group setting. A coach facilitates the program. In interactive lessons, student-athletes share goals and work together to improve their sport performance by learning how to eat better and train correctly.

ATLAS and ATHENA have undergone rigorous research evaluations and have been evaluated by numerous federal agencies for effectiveness, including the U.S. Department of Health and Human Services and the Government Accountability Office, the investigative arm of Congress.

and prevention materials targeted at anabolic steroids and other performance-enhancing drugs. The National Institute on Drug Abuse's Game Plan program, part of its Keep Your Body Healthy Campaign, seeks to encourage young men and women "to work with what nature has provided them"[72] rather than using steroids. The program includes public service announcements in English and Spanish, print ads, and posters. In 2009 the FDA extended its reach to include education about supplements, warning consumers to beware of any with androgen, estrogen, and progestin ingredients. The FDA commissioner says, "By pairing enforcement action with education, we hope to prevent others from being harmed by these products."[73]

A number of athletic organizations have included an anti-performance-enhancing drug component to their educational programs. The National Center for Drug Free Sport, which provides testing services for the NCAA, Major League Baseball's minor league program, and the Professional Golf Association tour, has a speakers' bureau and educational sessions targeted for athletes, coaches, and/or administrators. As part of its initiative to eliminate the use of performance-enhancing drugs among college athletes, the NCAA spends $800,000 annually on educational programs at colleges and universities. At the high school level, the National Federation of State High School Associations created a multimedia educational initiative called Make the Right Choice. In addition to educational materials targeting coaches and students, this program has materials designed for parents, who often underestimate the dangers of anabolic steroids and other performance-enhancing drugs.

Among the most successful educational programs for young people is the Athletes Training and Learning to Avoid Steroids (ATLAS) program, run by the Oregon Health and Science University (OHSU). The program specifically targets male athletes

Nine foreign governments assisted in Operation Raw Deal, the 2007 federal crackdown on illegal steroids. The operation led to more than 120 arrests and the seizure of 56 U.S. labs involved in illegal steroid manufacturing. Containers of steroids seized during the operation are pictured here.

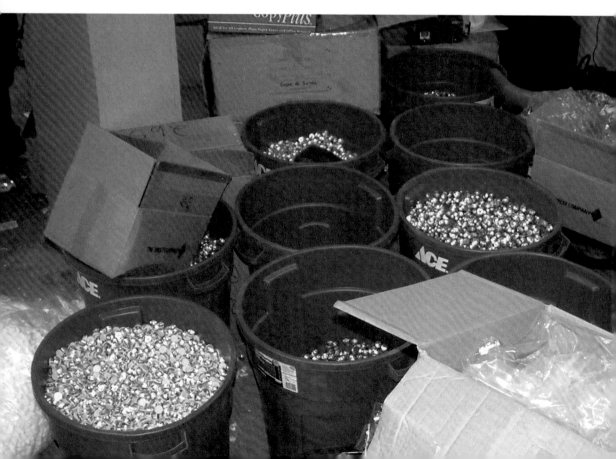

at the college level and includes multiple components to provide healthy sports nutrition and strength-training alternatives to the use of illicit and performance-enhancing drugs. At the core of the program are 10 peer-led, 45-minute sessions intended to be scheduled once a week during the season on a "light" practice day. OHSU conducts a similar program—Athletes Targeting Healthy Exercise and Nutrition Alternatives, or ATHENA—designed to meet the unique needs and issues of female athletes.

Athletes as Role Models

Some experts believe that the use of performance-enhancing substances among elite athletes may increase the risk that teens will follow in their footsteps. When young people hear that a successful athlete has used a drug with no ill effect, they may assume that the drug is safe—well before the long-term effects of using the drug can be known.

In recognition that young people want to do what their heroes do, antidrug campaigns have called on athletes as spokespersons. Athletes Against Steroids, for instance, was created in 2004 to fight the use of steroids by tapping drug-free athletes to serve as role models. The group's research, education, and outreach activities are designed to encourage young athletes to reject the pressure to use steroids and other illegal performance enhancers. The Web site provides information about the risks of steroid use, stories from ex-steroid users, and stories about deaths related to performance-enhancing drugs. A monthly newsletter provides information about how to achieve the same aims through nutrition, diet, and training. Major League Baseball has partnered with the Partnership for a Drug-Free America in a performance-enhancing drug awareness campaign. Several professional baseball players, including Derek Jeter, Jay Gibbons, Chipper Jones, and Kevin Millwood, have appeared in the campaign's TV and radio spots.

Hall of Fame linebacker Dick Butkus began the I Play Clean campaign to educate teens about the dangers of steroids. I Play Clean combines information about the risks of drugs with information about proper sports nutrition and "playing with attitude."[74] Butkus's program includes a long list of professional athletes, bodybuilders, and other celebrities who have vowed to stay away from drugs and asks students to take a pledge to join them.

Marion Jones is just one of many athletes who are sharing their stories of ruined lives. Through her Take a Break talk, which she plans to take to high schools nationwide, she hopes young people will learn from her mistakes. Jones's presentation begins with a short video showing highlights of her career and downfall. She then frankly discusses not only her poor choice of taking drugs, but also of lying to federal officials about her drug use. "I'm the one who decided to lie about using performance-enhancing drugs," she says frankly. "I am the one who decided to lie to myself because I was trying to avoid certain consequences. I lost my reputation. I suffered public humiliation."[75]

The Role of Parents and Coaches

Educators suggest that pressure for young athletes to succeed may contribute to the decision of some young people to take performance-enhancing drugs. Parents and coaches sometimes inadvertently add to the pressure of young people to succeed—and too often look the other way when they suspect a young athlete is using drugs. "The win-at-all-costs culture that pervades sports at all levels is a perfect incubator for cheating and the continued use of these dangerous substances," writes Bruce Svare. "Parents ignore the problem because they want their children to get an athletic scholarship or pro contract, even though they face long odds in realizing these goals."[76]

As part of their drug-prevention strategies, organizations often include materials targeting parents. "Our research confirms a genuine need to educate parents and teens about the risks of [steroids and performance-enhancing drugs]," says Steve Pasierb, president and CEO of the Partnership for a Drug-Free America. "Parents are critical in educating their kids about this dangerous category of drug abuse, but few believe their kids are at risk."[77] Educational materials for parents provide information about long-term health risks of drug use, what to look for to determine whether one's child is using performance-enhancing drugs, and strategies for preventing drug use.

Antidrug advocates also suggest that coaches play a pivotal role in an athlete's attitude toward drugs. The U.S. Department of Justice's Office of Juvenile Justice and Delinquency Prevention, for instance, has developed *The Coach's Playbook Against Drugs*. While this booklet is designed to engage coaches in discouraging drug use of any kind, its message is particularly relevant for performance-enhancing drugs. "It's important for coaches to take an active part in their players' lives—both on and off the field," says Darrell Green, a former defensive back for the Washington Redskins. "Positive role models are needed in our children's lives, and coaches have a special opportunity to deliver a powerful and consistent message about the dangers of drugs."[78]

Enhancing Effectiveness

Early attempts to prevent the illegal use of anabolic steroids among young people emphasized the risks of drug use. As with other drugs, such efforts have limitations. Research suggests that simply teaching students about the adverse effects of steroids does not convince adolescents that they personally can be adversely affected. In a 2008 survey, a majority of the students in grades 8 through 12 who admitted to using anabolic steroids said they would use a pill or a powder to reach their athletic goals, even if it would harm their health or shorten their life.

Research suggests that any discussion of the risks of performance enhancers should include not only the long-term health dangers but also the immediate impact that performance-enhancing drugs can have on the body and on athletic performance. Showing a young athlete how disrupted sleep—a side effect of anabolic steroids and many other drugs—can negatively impact reaction times and mental and physical agility, for instance, may help discourage drug use.

Studies suggest that young people may be more receptive to hearing about the dangers of drugs from peers than from adults. Peer counselors are a critical component of OHSU's highly effective ATLAS and ATHENA programs. Other young people who have had bad experiences with performance-enhancing drugs have

"Positive role models are needed in our children's lives, and coaches have a special opportunity to deliver a powerful and consistent message about the dangers of drugs."[78]

— Darrell Green, former professional football player.

told their stories through the news media or via the Internet. The Web site of the Taylor Hooton Foundation, which was created in memory of a 17-year-old teen athlete who took his own life after using steroids, provides testimony from a number of teens who have abused steroids.

Providing Alternatives

Preventing performance-enhancing drug abuse requires going beyond simply telling young people of the dangers of drug use. Effective programs address the root causes of drug use and provide alternatives. Pressures to perform well, to win, and to maintain their cool in the midst of intense training and competition are among the reasons athletes turn to drugs. Educators stress that successful drug-prevention programs need to address these pressures. Some programs provide team-building exercises in which athletes can discuss their pressures to perform.

Success depends on giving those at risk of using performance-enhancing drugs the tools they need to succeed without them. Effective programs show young people how to achieve these goals through more appropriate training techniques, such as diet and nutrition. Some programs also discuss how proper nutrition and strength training, including weight lifting, can help adolescents build their bodies without the use of drugs.

In some cases peers may play a role in encouraging a teen to try a performance-enhancing drug. It may be particularly hard for a student-athlete to turn down a drug if a team member suggests it will help the team succeed. Programs dealing with performance-enhancing drugs can be modeled after other antidrug programs, which teach young people how to deal with peer pressure and offer suggestions for how to reply when approached by someone offering a drug.

Given the wide range of reasons that people of all ages are tempted by performance-enhancing drugs, successful prevention will require a variety of prevention strategies reaching into various sectors of the community. Antidrug measures will have to reach far and wide into the population. Effective education and prevention programs will need to reach teens when they are first tempted to take a drug. These programs will also need to convince seasoned athletes that it is time to give the drugs up. A multipronged approach will be necessary to ensure that people understand that the risks—to one's health, career, and reputation—outweigh the benefits of using performance-enhancing drugs.

FACTS

- In one recent survey 40 percent of teens agreed that anabolic steroids are much safer to use than illegal drugs.

- An ongoing series of studies has shown that the multi-component, team-centered approach used by Oregon Health and Science University's Athletes Training and Learning to Avoid Steroids program reduces new steroid abuse by 50 percent.

- A 2008 survey published by the National Federation of State High School Associations shows that over 13 percent of high schools have a drug-testing policy in place; 63 percent of the schools drug test only student-athletes, and 20 percent test all students.

- In a 2007 survey 65 percent of colleges and universities reported that they have a drug/alcohol education program for student-athletes. This is 6 percent less than in 2005. These institutions indicated spending an average amount of $3,113 on drug education for student-athletes.

- In a 2009 survey undertaken in conjunction with the I Play Clean campaign, 85 percent of youths reported that they had never received education about steroids.

- In a 2008 survey of high school students, only 60 percent of those who were using anabolic steroids believed the drugs were dangerous. Nearly 60 percent of anabolic steroid users said they did not know that it was illegal to take the drugs without a prescription.

Related Organizations and Web Sites

Association Against Steroid Abuse

521 N. Sam Houston Pkwy. East, Suite 635
Houston, TX 77060
phone: (291) 999-9934
Web site: www.steroidabuse.com

The mission of the Association Against Steroid Abuse is to educate and safeguard against the abuse of anabolic steroids by providing information about and statistics on the dangers and issues relating to their use.

Athletes Against Steroids

731 Kirkman Rd.
Orlando, FL 32811
phone: (877) 914-9910
Web site: www.athletesagainststeroids.org

Athletes Against Steroids is an outreach and educational organization dedicated to eradicating steroids in sports.

National Center for Drug Free Sport

2537 Madison Ave.
Kansas City, MO 64108
phone: (816) 474-8655
fax: (816) 502-9287
Web site: www.drugfreesport.com

This organization provides drug-testing services and education programs. Clients include the National Collegiate Athletic Association, Major League Baseball's minor league program, the Professional Golf Association tour, and hundreds of universities and state high school associations and conferences.

National Coalition for the Advancement of Drug-Free Athletics (NCADFA)

PO Box 206
New Milford, NJ 07646
phone: (201) 265-8688
Web site: www.ncadfa.org

The NCADFA's purpose is to support educational, charitable, and scientific organizations engaged in antidrug education and prevention programs. The coalition also provides safe and effective alternatives to help athletes reach their potential.

National Collegiate Athletic Association (NCAA)

700 W. Washington St.
PO Box 6222
Indianapolis, IN 46206-6222
phone: (317) 917-6222
fax: (317) 917-6888
Web site: www.ncaa.org

The NCAA drug-testing program was created to protect the health and safety of student-athletes by ensuring that no participant has an artificially induced advantage or is pressured to use chemical substances.

Partnership for a Drug Free America

405 Lexington Ave., Suite 1601
New York, NY 10174
phone: (212) 922-1560
fax: (212) 922-1570
Web site: www.drugfreeamerica.org

The Partnership for a Drug-Free America provides education and awareness programs to prevent young people from using drugs, including performance-enhancing substances. Partnership materials also include a guide for parents and Coaches Corner, a blog about healthy sports for young people.

Taylor Hooton Foundation

PO Box 2104
Frisco, TX 75034-9998
phone: (972) 403-7300
Web site: www.taylorhooton.org

The Taylor Hooton Foundation for Fighting Steroid Abuse was formed in 2004 in memory of Taylor Hooton by his parents. Hooton was a high school athlete who took his own life at the age of 17 as a result of anabolic steroid abuse.

U.S. Anti-Doping Agency (USADA)

1330 Quail Lake Loop, Suite 260
Colorado Springs, CO 80906-4651
phone: (719) 785-2000
toll-free: (866) 601-2632
fax: (719) 785-2001
Web Site: www.usada.org

Founded in 2000, the USADA serves as the official anti-doping agency for Olympic-related sports in the United States and provides education and resources to deter the use of substances among athletes.

World Anti-Doping Agency (WADA)

800 Place Victoria, Suite 1700
Montreal, QC H4Z 1B7
Canada
phone: 1-514-904-9232
Web site: www.wada-ama.org.

WADA is an international independent agency composed of sports organizations and governments. It is involved in scientific research, education, development of drug tests and other anti-doping measures, and monitoring of prohibited substances and methods.

Additional Reading

Books

Shaun Assael, *Steroid Nation*. New York: ESPN, 2007.

S. Backhouse, J. McKenna, S. Robinson, and A. Atkin, *Attitudes, Behaviours, Knowledge and Education—Drugs in Sport: Past, Present and Future*. Montreal, QC: World Anti-Doping Agency, 2007.

José Canseco, *Vindicated: Big Names, Big Liars, and the Battle to Save Baseball*. New York: Simon Spotlight Entertainment, 2008.

Laura K. Egendorf, *Performance-Enhancing Drugs*. San Diego: ReferencePoint, 2007.

Mark S. Gold, *Performance-Enhancing Medications and Drugs of Abuse*. Binghamton, NY: Haworth Medical, 2007.

Thomas H. Murray, Karen J. Maschke, and Angela A. Wasunna, *Performance-Enhancing Technologies in Sports: Ethical, Conceptual, and Scientific Issues*. Baltimore: Johns Hopkins University Press, 2009.

Norah Piehl, *Performance-Enhancing Drugs*. Greenhaven, 2010.

Daniel M. Rosen, *Dope: A History of Performance Enhancement in Sports from the Nineteenth Century to Today*. Westport, CT: Praeger, 2008.

Teri Thomson, Nathaniel Vinton, Michael O'Keeffe, and Christian Red, *American Icon: The Fall of Roger Clemens and the Rise of Steroids in America's Pastime*. New York: Knopf, 2009.

Web Sites

Anabolic Steroid Abuse (www.steroidabuse.org). This National Institute on Drug Abuse Web site provides links to information and programs related to anabolic steroids and other performance-enhancing drugs.

"Are Steroids Worth the Risk?" Teens Health (www.kidshealth. org/teen/drug_alcohol/drugs/steroids.html). This Web site includes a wealth of articles and resources on steroid use by teens.

Drug Testing News (www.drugtestingnews.com). This Web site is designed to provide the most comprehensive source for up-to-date information on drug and alcohol testing, including legislation and technology.

National Institute on Drug Abuse, NIDA for Teens (http:// teens.drugabuse.gov/facts/facts_ster1.asp). This site includes basic steroid information for teens, including definitions, hormone information, and possible side effects on the teen body.

SteroidLaw.com. Sponsored by a lawyer who specializes in laws related to anabolic steroids and muscle-building dietary supplements, this Web site provides synopses of and links to news articles about steroid laws, proposed laws, and law enforcement activities.

Reports and Documents

National Institute on Drug Abuse, "Anabolic Steroid Abuse," Research Report Series. www.nida.nih.gov/ResearchReports/ Steroids/AnabolicSteroids.html.

World Anti-Doping Agency, *The World Anti-Doping Code: The 2010 Prohibited List, International Standard*, 2010. www. wada-ama.org/rtecontent/document/2010_Prohibited_List_ FINAL_EN_Web.pdf.

Source Notes

Introduction: A Growing Controversy

1. Quoted in Philippe Naughton, "Would-Be Marine Matthew Dear Died 'After Taking Steroids,'" *Times* (London), April 21, 2009. www.timesonline.co.uk.

2. Quoted in Millard Baker, "Death of Matthew Dear and Manufacturing Steroid Hysteria in the United Kingdom," *Iron Magazine,* April 28, 2009. www.ironmagazine.com.

3. Quoted in Baker, "Death of Matthew Dear and Manufacturing Steroid Hysteria in the United Kingdom."

4. Thomas H. Murray, "Sports Enhancement," Hastings Center, 2010. www.thehastingscenter.org.

Chapter One: What Are the Origins of the Performance-Enhancing Drugs Controversy?

5. David A. Baron, David M. Martin, and Samir Abol Magd, "Doping in Sports and Its Spread to At-Risk Populations: An International Review," *World Psychiatry*, June 2007. www.ncbi.nlm.nih.gov.

6. Quoted in John Hoberman, "Dopers on Wheels: The Tour's Sorry History," MSNBC, September 20, 2007. http://nbcsports.msnbc.com.

7. Quoted in Christine Brennan, "Babashoff Had Mettle to Speak Out About Steroids," *USA Today*, July 15, 2004. www.usatoday.com.

8. Quoted in Darren Beckham, "Blood Doping: Is It Really Worth It?" Texarkana College. www.tc.cc.tx.us.

9. Baron, Martin, and Magd, "Doping in Sports and Its Spread to At-Risk Populations."

10. Baron, Martin, and Magd, "Doping in Sports and Its Spread to At-Risk Populations."

11. John Hoberman, "Dopers on Wheels: The Tour's Sorry History," NBC Sports, September 20, 2007. http://nbcsports.msnbc.com.

12. Quoted in Hoberman, "Dopers on Wheels."

13. World Anti-Doping Agency, *The World Anti-Doping Code: The 2010 Prohibited List, International Standard*, September 19, 2009. www.wada-ama.org.

14. Quoted in Helen Branswell, "Experts Warn Gene Doping in Sport 'Inevitable' as Science Advances," MSN, February 4, 2010. http://news.ca.msn.com.

15. Quoted in Associated Press, "Bonds Moves into Eternity, Assumes MLB Home Run Record," ESPN, August 8, 2007. http://sports.espn.go.com.

16. Quoted in Anthony DiComo, "Selig: Report Is a Call to Action, " MLB, December 13, 2007. http://mlb.mlb.com.

17. Kristie Leong, "Teen Steroid Use: More Common than You Think," Associated Content, December 17, 2009. www.associatedcontent.com.

18. Nora D. Volkow, "Anabolic Steroid Abuse," National Institute on Drug Abuse, 2006. www.drugabuse.gov.

19. David Epstein, "Better Cycling Through Chemistry," *Guardian* (Manchester, UK), August 1, 2006. www.guardian.co.uk.

20. Quoted in Peter Handrinos, "Baseball Men: The Skeptic," Scout, December 18, 2006, http://stlcardinals.scout.com.

21. Quoted in Intelligence Squared, "We Should Accept Performance-Enhancing Drugs in Competitive Sports," January 15, 2008. http://intelligencesquaredus.org.

Chapter Two: Do Performance-Enhancing Drugs Pose a Health Risk?

22. Quoted in ESPN, "Drugs and Sports: Anabolic Steroids," September 6, 2007. http://espn.go.com.

23. National Institute on Drug Abuse, "Community Drug Alert Bulletin—Anabolic Steroids," April 2000. www.drugabuse.gov.

24. Quoted in Fox News, "Wrestler Chris Benoit Used Steroid Testosterone; Son Sedated Before Murders," July 17, 2007. www.foxnews.com.

25. Quoted in *Sports Illustrated*, "How We Got Here: A Time-line of Performance-Enhancing Drugs in Sports," March 11, 2008. http://sportsillustrated.cnn.com.

26. Quoted in Jeff Wilson, "Performance Enhancing Drugs Have Potentially Damaging Effects," *Observer*, January 28, 2005. http://observer.case.edu.

27. Quoted in Wilson, "Performance Enhancing Drugs Have Potentially Damaging Effects."

28. Quoted in Jennifer Thomas, "'Gene Doping' May Be Next Wave of Sports Tampering," MSN, February 4, 2010. http://health.msn.com.

29. Gary Cartwright, "Truth and Consequences," *Texas Monthly*, April 2008. www.texasmonthly.com.

30. Marylou Gantner, "I Know Where One Body Is—Still Fresh in the Grave," Athletes Against Steroids, 2004. www.athletesagainststeroids.org.

31. Quoted in Taylor Hooton Foundation, "Pete Kennedy," 2009. www.taylorhooton.org.

32. Kate Schmidt, "Just Say Yes to Steroids: Learn, Make Better Choices," *Nicholls Worth*, October 18, 2007. http://media.www.thenichollsworth.com.

Chapter Three: Do Performance-Enhancing Drugs Harm the Integrity of Sports?

33. Murray, "Sports Enhancement."

34. World Anti-Doping Agency, "Frequently Asked Questions," 2010. www.wada-ama.org.

35. Paul C. McCaffrey, "Playing Fair: Why the United States Anti-Doping Agency's Performance-Enhanced Adjudications

Should Be Treated as State Action," *Journal of Law & Politics*, 2006. https://litigation-essentials.lexisnexis.com.

36. Adrianne Blue, "It's the Real Dope," *New Statesman*, August 14, 2006. http://adrianneblue.com.

37. Quoted in Kevin Hayward, "Interview with *Steroid Nation* Author Gary Gaffney," All on the Field Sports Blog, November 28, 2007. http://allonthefield.blogspot.com.

38. Quoted in Jason Horowitz, "Linda McMahon, from Co-founder of the WWE to U.S. Senate Candidate," *Washington Post*, February 22, 2010. www.washingtonpost.com.

39. Quoted in *Sports Illustrated*, "McGwire Admits Steroid Use," January 11, 2010. http://sportsillustrated.cnn.com.

40. Jennifer Sey, "Let 'Em Eat Steroids," *Salon*, August 10, 2008. www.salon.com.

41. Sey, "Let 'Em Eat Steroids."

42. Quoted in Brian Biggane, "NFL Has Avoided Performance-Enhancing Drug Problems That Have Struck Baseball," *Palm Beach (FL) Post*, February 5, 2010. www.palmbeachpost.com.

43. Philip Wolf, "Fighting Drug Use by Elite Athletes Is Simply a Losing Battle," *Ottawa Citizen*, February 10, 2010. www.ottawacitizen.com.

44. Quoted in Roger Hensley, "Do Fans Really Care About PEDs?" STLtoday, July 2, 2009. http://interact.stltoday.com.

45. Jack Ewing, "Tour de France Raises Fresh Questions About Honesty in Sports," *Bloomberg Businessweek*, July 25, 2008. www.businessweek.com.

46. Quoted in Hayward, "Interview with *Steroid Nation* Author Gary Gaffney."

47. Timothy Noakes, "Should We Allow Performance-Enhancing Drugs in Sport? A Rebuttal to the Article by Savulescu and Colleagues," *International Journal of Sports Science and Coaching*, December 2006, p. 289.

48. Quoted in Hensley, "Do Fans Really Care About PEDs?"

49. Howard Bloom, "The National Football League and Performance-Enhancing Drugs (in Denial)," *Sports Business News*, September 12, 2006. http://sportsbiznews.blogspot.com.

50. Josh Millar, "The Best Punishment for Performance Enhancing Drugs: Make Them Legal," Bleacher Report, July 27, 2008. http://bleacherreport.com.

51. Quoted in Associated Press, "Jones Pleads Guilty, Admits Lying About Steroids," NBC Sports, October 5, 2007, p. 2. http://nbcsports.msnbc.com.

52. Quoted in ProCon.org, "Sports and Drugs: Historical Timeline," January 12, 2010. http://sportsanddrugs.procon.org.

53. Wolf, "Fighting Drug Use by Elite Athletes Is Simply a Losing Battle."

Chapter Four: Should Sports Organizations Take Stronger Measures to Stop Performance-Enhancing Drugs?

54. Quoted in George Spellwin, "Anabolic Steroid Testing: Texas Spends $6 Million and Catches 4 High School Students," Elite Fitness, February 23, 2009. http://bodybuilding.elitefitness.com.

55. Quoted in MSNBC, "Q&A: Impact of Steroids on Young Athletes," February 5, 2008. www.msnbc.msn.com.

56. Quoted in MSNBC, "Q&A."

57. Quoted in Stan Grossfield, "When Cheers Turn to Depression," *Boston Globe*, February 19, 2008. www.boston.com.

58. Quoted in Grossfield, "When Cheers Turn to Depression."

59. Spellwin, "Anabolic Steroid Testing."

60. Quoted in Drugstory, "Foul Play: Sports, Doping and Teens." www.drugstory.org.

61. Quoted in Amy Donaldson, "2010 Winter Olympics: IOC Is Winning War Against Doping," *Salt Lake City Deseret News*, February 27, 2010. www.deseretnews.com.

62. John Humphrys, "Let's Legalise Drugs in Sport and See What Happens," *Sunday Times* (London), October 26, 2003. www.timesonline.co.uk.

63. Quoted in Tom Reed and Mike Wagner, "When Hockey Playoffs Start, Drug Testing Stops," *Columbus (OH) Dispatch*, April 19, 2009. www.dispatch.com.

64. Quoted in Reed and Wagner, "When Hockey Playoffs Start, Drug Testing Stops."

65. Quoted in Reed and Wagner, "When Hockey Playoffs Start, Drug Testing Stops."

66. Quoted in *Talk of the Nation*, "Experts: 'Gene Doping' to Be Next Sports Scandal," National Public Radio, February 5, 2010. www.npr.org.

Chapter Five: How Can the Use of Performance-Enhancing Drugs Be Prevented?

67. Quoted in Associated Press, "Bill Requires Ingredients to Be Disclosed," ESPN, February 4, 2010. http://sports.espn.go.com.

68. Quoted in Senator John McCain Press Office, "Senator John McCain Introduces the Dietary Supplement Safety Act of 2010," February 3, 2010. http://mccain.senate.gov.

69. U.S. attorney's office, "Operation Phony Pharm: Six Charged as a Result of Investigation Targeting Internet Sale of Steroids, Human Growth Hormone," September 24, 2007. www.justice.gov.

70. Margaret A. Hamburg, "Remarks by Margaret A. Hamburg, M.D.," FDA, August 6, 2009. www.fda.gov.

71. Bruce Svare, "Solutions to Today's Sports Parenting Challenges," *Albany (NY) Times Union*, March 11, 2007. www.parentsforgoodsports.org.

72. National Institute on Drug Abuse, "Public Service Announcements: Keep Your Body Healthy." www.drugabuse.gov.

73. Hamburg, "Remarks by Margaret A. Hamburg, M.D."

74. Play Clean, "About Play Clean: Mission Statement." www.iplayclean.org.

75. Quoted in Maggie Jones, "What Makes Marion Jones Run?" *New York Times Magazine*, May 2, 2010, p. 36.

76. Svare, "Solutions to Today's Sports Parenting Challenges."

77. Quoted in Partnership for a Drug-Free America, "Major League Baseball Launches Anti-steroids Ad Campaign; Research-Based Effort Developed by the Partnership for a Drug-Free America," July 18, 2005. www.drugfree.org.

78. Quoted in U.S. Department of Justice Office of Juvenile Justice and Delinquency Prevention, *The Coach's Playbook Against Drugs*, p. 3. www.ncjrs.gov.

Index

About the Author

Lydia Bjornlund is a freelance writer. She has written more than 15 nonfiction books for children and teens, mostly on American history and health-related topics. She also writes books and training materials for adults on issues related to conservation and public management. Bjornlund holds a master's degree in education from Harvard University and a BA in American Studies from Williams College. She lives in northern Virginia with her husband, Gerry Hoetmer, and their children, Jake and Sophia.